T0298488

LIVING THERAPY SERIES

Counselling a Recovering Drug User

A Person-Centred Dialogue

Richard Bryant-Jefferies

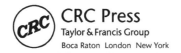

CRC Press
Taylor & Francis Group
Boca Raton London New York

CRC Press is an imprint of the
Taylor & Francis Group, an **informa** business

First published 2003 by Radcliffe Publishing

Published 2018 by CRC Press
Taylor & Francis Group
6000 Broken Sound Parkway NW, Suite 300
Boca Raton, FL 33487-2742

CRC Press is an imprint of Taylor & Francis Group, an Informa business

No claim to original U.S. Government works

ISBN-13: 978-1-85775-850-4 (pbk)

Visit the Taylor & Francis Web site at
http://www.taylorandfrancis.com

and the CRC Press Web site at
http://www.crcpress.com

British Library Cataloguing in Publication Data

A catalogue record for this book is available from the British Library.

Typeset by Aarontype Limited, Easton, Bristol

Contents

Foreword

The first thing that strikes me about this book is how readable it is. Usually when I read a book about a factual subject, in particular about medicine or other subjects related to my work, I tend to dip in and out over several weeks, as many textbooks I frankly find hard going. Not so with this book. I was riveted from the start as if I was reading a good novel.

Counselling a Recovering Drug User: a person-centred dialogue has a story line which gripped me like a magnet from cover to cover. By the time I had read the book not only had I gained an insight into a drug user's life and the complicated issues that can affect them, but I also felt that I had had a damned good read. I had also learned about the principles behind Rogerian person-centred counselling and some of the issues which may confront both the client and the therapist within this type of encounter. Throughout the book Richard Bryant-Jefferies manages to put across these issues, whilst at the same time gripping the reader in the story line.

Another important part of the process is that of supervision of the therapist. The reader will not only see that supervision is a desirable facility for a health worker but is an essential element in supporting the worker and encouraging critical analysis and thus deeper understanding of the relationship and dynamics of the encounter. Having worked as a doctor for 22 years without ever receiving any formal supervision, after reading this book I feel slightly lacking and quite let down as the benefits are shown so eloquently in this book, not only for the therapist, but also for the therapeutic process itself.

Aside from certainly enjoying this book, the reader will come away with a heightened awareness and increased knowledge of the complexities of dealing with people who have a drug-related problem. Richard Bryant-Jefferies evidently has a deep understanding himself and is able to communicate these issues in an easy-to-understand way, at the same time stimulating but not taxing the reader's mind. Within the story line are inset boxes in which the author provides the reader with a commentary on the counselling process and explains some of the practicalities of drug using, thereby giving a greater depth to the reading experience. At the end of each chapter there is a useful summary and a list of points for discussion which encourage the reader to become involved in the counselling process and the issues which both the client and counsellor encounter.

Many people will benefit from this book. The lay reader will find the book an engaging read whilst gaining some insight into the world of drug users and the counselling process. Actual and potential clients may read this and gain encouragement about the benefits of person-centred counselling. Health professionals will find this book provides an easy-to-follow explanation of Carl Rogers' counselling model and a unique view on how the counselling relationship allows a troubled client to grow and heal.

Anyone reading this book will not fail to notice Richard Bryant-Jefferies' non-judgemental approach to the drug user, which is essential if any therapeutic relationship is to work. They will also not fail to question their own judgement of other human beings in light of the author's humbling respect for others.

I enjoyed this book immensely. If other textbooks were as easy to read I would have a much greater knowledge and a deeper understanding of many subject areas. As with his earlier book, *Problem Drinking: a person-centred approach*, Richard Bryant-Jefferies has a winner. I highly recommend this book to anyone who has an interest in drug users' problems and the therapeutic relationship.

Dr Peter C Robinson MB, BS, DRCOG
General Practitioner, Farnham, Surrey
GP with a Special Interest in Substance Misuse, Guildford, Surrey
Hospital Practitioner in Genito-Urinary Medicine, Guildford, Surrey
GP Tutor, St George's Hospital Medical School, London
August 2003

Foreword

In the past decade, research has overwhelmingly established that drug abuse and drug dependence is a disorder with symptoms that manifest themselves in all aspects of life. It is no longer acceptable for anyone to view a person who has a drug abuse problem as a matter of a person being morally deficient and lacking sufficient amounts of willpower to change behavior. Persons with drug abuse disorders are also on the rise according to recent reports from the Global Burden of Disease and the World Health Organization. It is estimated 141 million people worldwide are drug abusers. Recent data from the UK Department of Health estimate the social and economic costs of drug use in the UK at £4 billion a year. Drug-related deaths have continued to rise in England, Wales, Scotland and Northern Ireland. These numbers have a significant impact on individuals, families and communities at local, national and international levels in relation to public health problems associated with drug abuse.

Richard Bryant-Jefferies' book is well timed and critically needed because it is a unique focus specifically working with the individual drug abuser which is written within the framework of Carl Rogers' person-centered approach. Why is this important? It is important because for far too long it has been a belief in the drug treatment field that persons having drug problems are in denial due to personality deficits, and are immoral. A mainstay of treatment has been aggressive confrontation treatments which may demoralize a person and attempt to coerce positive behavioral changes. Counseling behaviors, however, using such approaches have been shown to predict treatment failure. An almost exact opposite approach, use of empathy, has been associated with successful outcomes of treatment. Humanistic approaches have been utilized for other psychological problems for a number of years but very few times have these approaches been used when treating a person for drug abuse.

In a classic paper in 1936, Rosenzwiez introduced the concept of common factors. Common factors are not specifically unique interventions or approaches used but are factors, such as warmth, attention, understanding, and encouragement, which are central to, and play an active role in, client improvement. Project Match, a study in the USA, supported evidence of the importance of these types of common factors as criteria for success for persons treated for addiction problems. Project Match studied outcomes of persons who were substance dependent and found that all patients who participated in the study showed sustained, significant improvement with positive outcomes. The improved outcomes were found to be related to the high quality of care each person perceived they were receiving, not one of the three different behavioral approaches used in the study. Other recent studies support the effectiveness of a therapist's style using empathy with successful client outcomes. Furthermore, regardless of the treatment technique used by a counselor, the counselors who create a strong therapeutic alliance and relationship with their client have better improvement outcomes for the client.

Bryant-Jefferies' book, *Counselling a Recovering Drug User: a person-centred dialogue*, does exactly this. This book is matchless and deeply insightful. It brings alive the work formulated by Carl Rogers in defining and utilizing the necessary and sufficient conditions, which Bryant-Jefferies demonstrates, to bring positive behavioral life-style changes for a person experiencing a drug problem. Bryant-Jefferies offers critical wisdom from his many years of counseling persons with substance abuse problems and brings into the text the guidance and skill of an experienced supervisor. This in turn offers counseling suggestions, which are within reach for all who read this book. The therapeutic alliance at work within the pages of this book describes brilliantly the relationship of three people working together, the client, the counselor and the counselor's supervisor, to actively improve the life of one person struggling with a drug problem.

No doubt Bryant-Jefferies' book will remain a reference for a long time to come for all of us working in the field of counseling persons with drug abuse problems.

Dana Murphy-Parker RN, MS, CNS
Professor of Nursing, Arizona Western College
Board of Directors, The International Nurses Society on Addictions
Chair, Education Committee
The International Network of Nurses (TINN) Interested in Alcohol
Co-Founder, Tobacco and Drug Misuse
August 2003

Preface

Few general counselling training courses include a great deal on the subject of working with people with drug problems. Yet counsellors and other health and social care professionals are being faced with clients who, for one reason or another, have developed a drug-using habit, or may have had one in the past and may still be carrying the effects of drug use. The counsellor in the GP surgery, the nurse in the accident and emergency department, the social worker concerned with a family, the housing support worker in a city centre hostel can all expect to encounter people with drug problems. In fact, the list is endless: drug use is so widespread these days that you are likely to encounter it anywhere and everywhere.

I am aware of the growing need for a wider understanding of the issues to be addressed and ways of working with this client group if we are to ensure that damage is minimised, both to the user and to others. There is so much prejudicial and judgemental thought around in relation to this group of people, and I hope that this book will help to emphasise that the drug user is more, much more, than their drug use. The client in this book is not a stereotype; recovering drug users are individual with their own set of experiences and meanings that they attribute to their drug use.

This book sets out to provide material to inform the training process of counsellors and many others who seek to work with this client group. It is intended as much for experienced counsellors as it is for trainees. It provides real insight into what can occur during counselling sessions where the client is seeking to resolve issues related to their drug use, reflection on the process, and helpful summaries and points for discussion in the wide range of training courses for which it is intended.

Counselling a Recovering Drug User: a person-centred dialogue will also be of value to the many healthcare and social care professionals who are likely to encounter patients or clients, or relatives of these, with this kind of problem. For all these professionals, the text demystifies what can occur in therapy, and at the same time provides useful approaches and frameworks that may be used by professionals other than counsellors.

Importantly, I have also written this book for the person who has thought of seeking help for issues underlying their drug use, offering them insight into the process that they might expect in order to resolve their difficulty. However, one book can only convey part of the story. There may be common factors, but essentially each person is unique, using substances for their own reasons. These need to be recognised and understood, with the client being offered the therapeutic environment and relationship which promote constructive personality change.

There are perhaps as many myths about counselling as there are about drug use. I hope that this book helps to reveal to readers the role of the sensitive and supportive counsellor in working with a person who has a long history of drug use, itself a symptom of deeper, traumatic experiences.

Richard Bryant-Jefferies
August 2003

About the author

Richard Bryant-Jefferies qualified in person-centred counselling in 1994 and remains passionate about the application and effectiveness of this approach. From early 1995 he has worked at a community drug and alcohol service in Surrey. As well as having experience of offering counselling within this specialist arena, he has also supervised counsellors who work with people with drug and alcohol problems, has worked himself as a general counsellor in a GP surgery and offers general counselling supervision. He also offers training in working with people who have alcohol problems. Richard has recently accepted a new role as a manager of substance misuse services in London.

Richard has had articles published in journals (including *CPJ*, *HCPJ*, *Practice Nurse*) and had his first book on a counselling theme published in 2001, *Counselling the Person Beyond the Alcohol Problem* (Jessica Kingsley Publishers), providing theoretical yet practical insights into the application of the person-centred approach within the context of the 'cycle of change' model that has been widely adopted to describe the process of change.

Since then he has been writing for the *Living Therapy* series, producing an on-going series of person-centred dialogues: *Problem Drinking*, *Time Limited Therapy in Primary Care* and *Counselling a Survivor of Child Sexual Abuse*.

Richard is keen to bring the experience of the therapeutic process, from the standpoint and application of the person-centred approach, to a wider audience. He is convinced that the attitudinal values of this approach and the emphasis it places on the therapeutic relationship are key to helping people resolve not just problematic drug use, but the issues that generally lie beneath it, fuelling the urge to use.

Acknowledgements

I would like to express my gratitude to the following professionals who contributed helpful and insightful feedback on the draft for this book: Pauline Redgrift, a person-centred counsellor and drug worker, and Nadine Page, who manages an NHS GP liaison alcohol service.

I would also like to thank the series editor, Maggie Pettifer, for her continued encouragement towards the writing of the *Living Therapy* series. I know that she, like me, heartily believes in the significance of this style of presenting person-centred counselling applied to specific contexts and experiences.

Introduction

In many ways this book is probably unique insofar as it is written to offer the reader an opportunity to experience and to appreciate some of the diverse and challenging issues that can arise when working with a person who has had, and is struggling with, a drug problem. It is composed almost totally of dialogue between a fictitious client (Dan) and his counsellor (Jeannie), and between the counsellor and her supervisor (Max). Within the dialogue are woven the reflective thoughts and feelings of the client, the counsellor and the supervisor.

The dialogue has been written with the aim of demonstrating Jeannie's application of the Person-Centred Approach (PCA) – a theoretical approach to counselling that has, at its heart, the power of the relational experience to offer the client an experience through which greater potential for authentic living may emerge. The approach is widely used by counsellors working in the UK today: in a membership survey in 2001 by the British Association for Counselling and Psychotherapy, 35.6 per cent of those responding claimed to work to the person-centred approach, while 25.4 per cent identified themselves as psychodynamic practitioners.

The reader may find that it takes a while to adjust to the dialogue format. Many of the responses offered by Jeannie are reflections of what Dan has said. This is not to be read as conveying a simple repetition of the client's words. Rather, the counsellor seeks to voice empathic responses, often with a sense of 'checking out' that she is hearing accurately what the client is saying. The client says something; the counsellor then conveys that she has heard it, sometimes with the same words, sometimes including a sense of what she feels may be being communicated through the client's tone of voice, facial expression or simply the atmosphere of the moment. The client is then enabled to confirm that he has been heard accurately, or correct the counsellor in her perception. The client may then explore more deeply what he has been saying or move on, in either case with a sense that he has been heard and warmly accepted. To draw this to the reader's attention, I have attempted to highlight some of the reflections that occur throughout the work by inserting Jeannie's reflective thoughts in boxes throughout the dialogue.

The four supervision sessions are included to offer the reader insight into the nature of therapeutic supervision in the context of the counselling profession, a method of supervising that I term 'collaborative review'. For many trainee counsellors, the use of supervision can be something of a mystery, and it is hoped that this book will go a long way towards unravelling this. In the supervision sessions I seek to demonstrate the application of the supervisory relationship. My intention is to show how supervision of the counsellor is very much a part of the process of enabling a client to work through issues that in this case relate to the client's drug use.

Many professions do not recognise the need for some form of personal and process supervision, and often what is offered is line management. However, counsellors are required to receive regular supervision in order to explore the dynamics of the relationship with the client, the impact of the work on the counsellor and on the client, to receive support and to provide an opportunity for an experienced co-professional to monitor the supervisee's work in relation to ethical standards and codes of practice. The supervision sessions are included because they are an integral part of the therapeutic process. It is also hoped that they will help readers from other professions to recognise the value of some form of supportive and collaborative supervision in order to help them become more authentically present with their own clients.

I also favour an approach that is of a collaborative nature which I tend to describe as a process of 'collaborative review'. Merry (2002) describes what he terms as 'collaborative inquiry' as a 'form of research or inquiry in which two people (the supervisor and the counsellor) collaborate or co-operate in an effort to understand what is going on within the counselling relationship and within the counsellor'. There are, of course, as many models of supervision as there are models of counselling. In this book the supervisor is seeking to apply the attitudinal values of the person-centred approach.

It is the norm for all professionals working in the healthcare and social care environment in this age of regulation to be formally accredited or registered and to work to their own professional organisation's code of ethics or practice. For instance, registered counselling practitioners with the British Association for Counselling and Psychotherapy are required to have regular supervision and continuing professional development to maintain registration. While professionals other than counsellors will gain much from this book in their work with patients or clients with drug-related problems, it is essential that they follow the standards, safeguards and ethical codes of their own professional organisation, and are appropriately trained and supervised to work with their clients.

All characters in this book are fictitious and are not intended to bear resemblance to any particular person or persons.

The person-centred approach

The person-centred approach (PCA) was formulated by Carl Rogers, and references are made to his ideas within the text of the book. However, it will be helpful for readers who are unfamiliar with this way of working to have an appreciation of its theoretical base.

Rogers proposed that certain conditions, when present within a therapeutic relationship, would enable the client to develop towards what he termed 'fuller functionality'. Over a number of years he refined these ideas, which he defined as 'the necessary and sufficient conditions for constructive personality change'. These he described as follows.

1 Two persons are in psychological contact.
2 The first, whom we shall term the client, is in a state of incongruence, being vulnerable or anxious.
3 The second person, whom we shall term the therapist, is congruent or integrated in the relationship.
4 The therapist experiences unconditional positive regard for the client.
5 The therapist experiences an empathic understanding of the client's internal frame of reference and endeavours to communicate this experience to the client.
6 The communication to the client of the therapist's empathic understanding and unconditional positive regard is to a minimal degree achieved (Rogers, 1957, p.96).

The first necessary and sufficient condition given for constructive personality change is that of 'two persons being in psychological contact'. However, although he later published this as simply 'contact' (Rogers, 1959), it is suggested (by Wyatt and Sanders, 2002, p.6) that this was actually written in 1953–54. They quote Rogers as defining contact in the following terms: 'Two persons are in psychological contact, or have the minimum essential relationship, when each makes a perceived or subceived difference in the experiential field of the other' (Rogers, 1959, p.207). A recent exploration of the nature of psychological contact from a person-centred perspective is given by Warner (2002).

Rogers defined empathy as meaning 'entering the private perceptual world of the other ... being sensitive, moment by moment, to the changing felt meanings which flow in this other person ... It means sensing meanings of which he or she is scarcely aware, but not trying to uncover totally unconscious feelings' (1980, p.142). It is a very delicate process, and it provides, I believe, a foundation block. The counsellor's role is primarily to establish empathic rapport and communicate empathic understanding to the client.

Within this relationship the counsellor seeks to maintain an attitude of unconditional positive regard towards the client and all that they disclose. This is not 'agreeing with', it is simply warm acceptance. Rogers wrote, 'when the therapist is experiencing a positive, acceptant attitude towards whatever the client *is* at that moment, therapeutic movement or change is more likely to occur (1980, p.116). Mearns and Thorne suggest that:

'unconditional positive regard is the label given to the fundamental attitude of the person-centred counsellor towards her client. The counsellor who holds this attitude deeply values the humanity of her client and is not deflected in that valuing by any particular client behaviours. The attitude manifests itself in the counsellor's consistent acceptance of and enduring warmth towards her client' (Mearns and Thorne, 1988, p.59).

Last, but by no means least, is that state of being that Rogers referred to as congruence, but which has also been described in terms of 'realness', 'transparency', 'genuineness', 'authenticity'. Indeed Rogers wrote that '. . . genuineness, realness or congruence . . . this means that the therapist is openly being the feelings and attitudes that are flowing within at the moment. The term "transparent" catches the flavor of this condition' (Rogers, 1980, p. 115). Putting this into the therapeutic setting, we can say that 'congruence is the state of being of the counsellor when her outward responses to her client consistently match the inner feelings and sensations which she has in relation to her client' (Mearns and Thorne, 1999, p.84).

I would suggest that any congruent expression by the counsellor of their feelings or reactions has to emerge through the process of being in therapeutic relationship with the client. It is a disciplined response and not an open door to endless self-disclosure. Congruent expression is perhaps most appropriate and therapeutically valuable where it is informed by the existence of an empathic understanding of the client's inner world, and is offered in a climate of a genuine warm acceptance towards the client.

PCA regards the relationship that we have with our clients, and the attitude that we hold within that relationship, to be key factors. In my experience, many adult psychological difficulties develop out of life experiences that involve problematic, conditional or abusive relational experiences. This can be centred in childhood or later in life. What is significant is that the individual, through relationships that have a negative conditioning effect, is left with a distorted perception of themselves and their potential as a person. I see many people who have learned from childhood experience beliefs such as 'I can never be good enough to be praised for what I have achieved; I never match my parents' expectations' or 'No one was ever there for me when I was hurting; perhaps I am unlovable'. The result is a loss of a positive sense of self, and the individual adapts to maintain the newly learned concept of self. This is then lived out, possibly throughout life, the person seeking to satisfy what they have come to believe about themselves: being unable to achieve, feeling unable or undeserving to be loved, though perhaps in both cases maintaining a constant desperation to receive what they never had. Yet, perversely, they may then sabotage any possibility of gaining what they want in order to maintain the negatively conditioned sense of self and the sense of satisfaction that this gives them because they have developed such a strong identity with it.

It is my belief that by offering someone a non-judgemental, warm and accepting, and authentic relationship, the person can grow into a fresh sense of self in which their potential as a person can become more fulfilled. Such an experience fosters an opportunity for the client to redefine themselves as they experience the presence of the therapist's congruence, empathy and unconditional positive regard. This process can take time. Often the personality change that is required to sustain a shift away from what have been termed 'conditions of worth' requires a lengthy period of therapeutic work, bearing in mind that the person may be struggling to unravel a sense of self that has been developed, sustained and reinforced for many decades of life.

The term 'conditions of worth' applies to the conditioning that is frequently present in childhood, and at other times in life, when a person experiences that their worth is conditional on their doing something, or behaving, in a certain way. This is usually to satisfy someone else's needs, and can be contrary to the client's own sense of what would be a satisfying experience. The values of others become a feature of the individual's structure of self. The person moves away from being true to themselves, learning instead to remain 'true' to their conditioned sense of worth. This state of being in the client is challenged by the person-centred therapist by offering them unconditional positive regard and warm acceptance. Such a therapist, by genuinely offering these therapeutic attitudes, provides the client with an opportunity to be exposed to what may be a new experience or one that in the past they have dismissed, preferring to stay with that which matches and therefore reinforces their conditioned sense of worth and sense of self. Unconditional positive regard and warm acceptance offered consistently over time can, and does, enable clients to begin to question their beliefs about themselves and to begin to build into their structure of self the capacity to see and experience themselves as being of value for who they are. It enables them to liberate themselves from the constraints of patterns of conditioning.

A crucial feature or factor in this process is the presence of what Rogers termed 'the actualising tendency', a tendency towards fuller and more complete personhood with an associated greater fulfilment of their potentialities. The role of the person-centred counsellor is to provide the facilitative climate within which this tendency can work constructively. The 'therapist trusts the actualizing tendency of the client and truly believes that the client who experiences the freedom of a fostering psychological climate will resolve his or her own problems' (Bozarth, 1998, p.4). This is fundamental to the application of the person-centred approach. Rogers (1986, p.198) wrote:

'the person-centred approach is built on a basic trust in the person ... (It) depends on the actualizing tendency present in every living organism – the tendency to grow, to develop, to realize its full potential. This way of being trusts the constructive directional flow of the human being towards a more complex and complete development. It is this directional flow that we aim to release.'

The therapeutic relationship is central. A therapeutic approach such as person-centred affirms that it is not what you do so much as *how you are* with your client that is therapeutically significant, and this 'how you are' has to be received by the client. Gaylin (2001, p.103) highlights the importance of client perception. 'If clients believe that their therapist is working on their behalf – if they perceive caring and understanding – then therapy is likely to be successful. It is the condition of attachment and the perception of connection that have the power to release the faltered actualization of the self.' He goes on to stress how 'we all need to feel connected, prized – loved', describing human beings as 'a species born into mutual interdependence', and that there 'can be no self outside the context of others. Loneliness is dehumanizing and isolation anathema to the human condition.' 'The relationship', he suggests, 'is what psychotherapy is all about.'

There is currently growing interest in, and much debate about, theoretical developments within the person-centred world and its application. Discussions on the theme of Rogers' therapeutic conditions presented by various key members of the person-centred community have recently been published (Bozarth and Wilkins, 2001; Haugh and Merry, 2001; Wyatt, 2001; Wyatt and Sanders, 2002). It seems to me that the relational component of the person-centred approach, based on the presence of the core conditions, is emerging strongly as a counter to the sense of isolation that frequently accompanies deep psychological and emotional problems, and the increase in what I would term a 'rabid inauthenticity' within materialistic societies as we enter the twenty-first century.

This is obviously a very brief introduction to the approach. Person-centred theory continues to develop as practitioners and theoreticians consider its application in various fields of therapeutic work and extend our theoretical understanding of developmental and therapeutic processes. At times it feels like it has become more than just individuals; rather it feels like a group of colleagues, based around the world, working together to penetrate deeper towards a more complete theory of the human condition. It is an exciting time.

Drug use

First of all, we need to clarify some definitions. Are drugs used, or abused, or misused? This may seem an absurd question and many people will react to it by saying, 'Well, it's drug abuse; the person is abusing a substance, and abusing their bodies as well.' But is it that simple? We all make choices to do things in order to gain an experience: a thrill, to feel better, to get away from discomfort. Is the decision to use a drug to achieve this anything other than another choice? Well, yes, but also no, because of the chemically addictive nature of some substances, but not all. Some are not chemically addictive, but they are psychologically addictive, leaving the person experiencing a dramatic need to re-experience some psychological state, or to enable them to achieve a particular mood in order to deal with some issue or situation arising in life, or escape from it. We make choices in order to experience something and generally to experience something that is better than that which existed before the choice was made. 'Changes do not come easily unless one has a reason to want to change, and even then it can be hard to break out of familiar habits. When we know a particular experience makes us feel "good" or "better" or "normal", it is difficult not to repeat it' (Bryant-Jefferies, 2002, p.175).

We use food to feel comfortable. So, if we overeat – comfort eating, often involving a lot of sugar – which may lead to health problems, does that mean we indulge in 'food abuse'? We may go to the gym to feel good, make our bodies feel alive. But if we become addicted to going to the gym because of endorphine release and the mood lift it gives us, and we are spending time there which should be given to other matters, are we experiencing 'gym abuse'? Or we may like the camaraderie and sense of belonging by being part of a group having a distinctive identity. If we spend our lives following a football team to the point that money is spent on that rather than meeting other basic family needs, are we suffering from 'football abuse'? These are not terms we generally use, and yet the person who overuses a chemical, seeks a chemical to feel more alive, or spends money on chasing the chemical rather than on household needs is called a 'drug abuser'. In the final analysis, all we have is a choice that causes a problem. But the complicating factor is, of course, that many mood-altering drugs are illicit (except those prescribed, although these also find their way on to the streets as we know). Tyler (1995, p.11) offers the view that 'someone who binges daily on cup cakes and sugary tea is being more self-destructive than a once a month moderate heroin snorter'.

So what about the term 'misuse', which is also often applied to drug use. Does the person misuse the substance? To misuse something is in effect to use it for a purpose other than that for which it was created. Most designer drugs are created for the purpose of giving someone a psychological experience, or to give them more energy, or relax them, and these are the reasons for which they are used. Organic drugs such as cannabis and heroin have certain effects on a person's experiencing, and are chosen in order to achieve that experience. But then so is caffeine in coffee, or sugar in cakes and biscuits, or cocoa in chocolate. So are these substances being 'misused'? Yet again, probably not.

We are left then with 'use'. Drug use. Drug users. The reality is that people use drugs to gain an experience, and then either continue chasing that same experience, or the addictive nature of the drug means they have to keep using it simply to stave off withdrawal reactions which can be extremely unpleasant and, for a drug such as alcohol, can be life-threatening.

A wide range of people use drugs; it crosses the social and economic spectrum. And it is a growing issue and a growing problem as more and more young people experiment with, and are drawn into, addictive habits that then generate further problems. But not for everyone. Many drug users will manage to maintain their use at a recreational level. They will remain 'drug users'. They will not be dependent, not use to the point at which they may need to thieve or deal, or prostitute their bodies to get money to pay for their habits.

However, there will be a large number of people for whom these activities become their daily reality as they struggle to maintain their habit, or people for whom habitual drug use generates difficulties in their lives: loss of job, accidents, mental and physical health problems. By definition, we can classify this group as 'problem drug users': their drug use is associated with or generates problems of one kind or another.

So we have *drug users* and *problem drug users*; it is as simple as that.

Problem drug users will tend to evidence chaotic lives. Increasingly, people who use drugs tend to use more than one type – becoming 'polydrug users'. Their drug use has become central in their lives, possibly to the detriment of anything and everything else. Working with a client who is at the problematic

stage will generate huge challenges: they may be inconsistent in their atten-
dance; they may attend drug-affected; they will be engaging, perhaps, in risky
behaviour in terms of injecting practices, mixing substances, risking overdose by
using street drugs whose strength may be unknown. Life has become drug-
centred, and their mission in life, it can seem, is simply to obtain the next hit.
Problem drug users can find themselves living for their drugs.

However, let us not forget that the problem drug user is a person, like you and
me, a human being with thoughts and feelings and needs. If this is your belief,
then like us they will have a spirit, whatever that may mean to you. The drug
user hurts, she bleeds, he has tears. Yet we can so easily lose sight of this. The
person-centred approach argues the importance of acknowledging and reaching
out to the person who is using the drugs. Within the chaos of behaviours associated with problematic drug use exists a person, doing the best they can to
survive, possibly carrying with them a whole host of difficult and painful experiences, many traumatic, which may not have initially caused the choice to use
drugs (though often it can have) but which are now being dealt with by maintaining drug-induced states of mind and feeling. Can we, as counsellors, reach into
the chaos and seek to let our drug-using client know that we see their personhood? If we cannot, or are not prepared to do this, then we need to work with a
different client group.

Problem drug users are often described as devious, manipulative, not to be
trusted. Anyone who is addicted to something will seek that something out and,
if the addiction is strong enough, at any cost. The allure of the drug-induced state,
or the need to avoid the discomfort of withdrawal, ensures that the individual will
be urged on by a primary drive to obtain their drug(s) of choice.

Yet not all who use drugs do so in a problematic way, in the same way that not
everyone who drinks alcohol does so in a problematic manner, or to problematic
effect. There are many, many people who *use* drugs, and their use does not generate for them or for those around them a problem – other than if it is an illegal
drug then they may experience legal problems if caught. But people can safely
use some substances in such a way as to minimise harmful effects; people can
and do use substances recreationally and not experience health problems or find
themselves evidencing problematic behaviours.

However, a difficulty we face is with the long-term effects of substance use
when that use begins at an early age when the individual is still developing.
Only over time will we understand the long-term organic impact, and what impli-
cation this will have for both physical and mental health. And we must not forget
emotional health and psychological development. Sharing needles increases the
risk of infection, in particular of HIV and hepatitis. Brain chemistry can be
affected,   with some substances leaving people with long-term problems:
racing thoughts, depression, paranoia, psychotic episodes. Added to this, in my
experience, early substance use can and does affect a person's ability to develop
emotionally, leaving them in later life with the body of an adult but the feelings
and often the thought processing of a teenager, or even a younger child.

There are many explanations for drug use. Carr (2002, pp.590–694) offers
seven broad theoretical categories. First, 'Biological Theory', which includes

genetic factors, temperament and a tendency to risk taking, and the development of or predisposition towards tolerance and dependence. Next, 'Intrapsychic Deficit Theories', which include stress and the development of coping strategies, for instance with early life trauma, but are also linked to dealing with the psychological and emotional impact of academic failure. He also includes here drug use as a means for the individual striving for autonomy, their own life, distinct from perhaps parental or social norms.

Under the title of 'Behavioural Theories' he includes positive reinforcement through achieved mood change and later more negative conditioning linked to avoiding withdrawal experiences. Also to be considered here is what he terms 'classical conditioning', such as exposures to cues and triggers that are associated with drug use. This brings us to another range of factors, those linked to 'Family Systems Theories', where parental drug use, parenting styles and family disorganisation are highlighted as significant factors.

We can then extend to factors beyond the family, to 'Sociological Theories', which include social disadvantage, a sense of alienation from societal values, the availability of drugs and the culture of drug use as a social norm, for instance within a given geographical or demographic area.

Another theoretical group is that of 'Multiple Risk Factors'. This is where a number of the risk factors already alluded to are present. It seems reasonable to suggest that the more risk factors that are present, the greater the likelihood of that individual using drugs, and perhaps where the risk factors present involve greater chaos, unpredictability and uncertainty in the life of the individual, then the individual so affected in early life may develop a pattern of drug use that tends more towards being problematic.

A final grouping that Carr offers is that made up of 'Theories of Recovery and Relapse', which includes the theories about the nature of the process of change and of relapse processes.

In reading through this book you will note that many of these factors have been present within the client's life experience, and have become contributory triggers to his own developing drug use.

Setting the scene

This book deals with working with a drug user, someone who has experienced problems associated with drug use but who is trying to break free of it. The client has been a user of many different substances, including opiates, and he is currently on a methadone script, a substitute opiate prescribed widely as a harm-minimisation strategy to break the cycle of injecting and to create a more stable basis for further reduction in use where this is felt to be a realistic goal by the client.

The client has been referred for counselling as part of his process of addressing and resolving underlying issues, many of which are likely to be associated with his drug use. This follows his chemical stabilisation. He is also seen by a

keyworker at the clinic he attends, and a doctor who is responsible for prescribing his methadone on a weekly basis. The clinic does not offer daily pick-up and
supervised consumption except for extremely chaotic clients. In this case the
client has achieved stability and is trusted with his week's supply.

The client has had a number of years of chaotic drug use. This, together with
the difficult childhood experiences that he describes, has left him with a tendency
towards wanting to maintain some degree of chaos. It is not unusual. It presents a
huge challenge to counsellors. This tendency to chaos can re-emerge, and seemingly at any time. Drugs are powerful and, with all the motivation in the
world, clients can lapse back into old patterns of use, only to return to a service
worse than when they left. The counsellor may find that their offering of warm
acceptance, empathic understanding and an authentic presence is simply not
enough to contain the urge to use. And once under the influence of the drugs
the person may break contact and it could be weeks, months, years before they
return for help.

So counselling a drug user is a risky business. Anything can happen, and
happen fast. The counsellor must have regular supervision that meets both her
professional and personal needs. 'Containment of clients in chaos may be the
best we can do, paying attention to their crisis whilst not becoming chaotic ourselves, and using our supervision to "hold" us. In supervision I am able to regain
perspective and make sense of what has happened' (Bedor, 2002, p.196).

The following pages offer a window into the world of counselling the recovering drug user, providing insight into some of the issues that can arise and how,
from a person-centred perspective, the counsellor may respond. The counsellor is
not demonstrating perfection; she makes mistakes, misses things, gets in the way
of the client and does all the things that counsellors can do because they are not
perfect. But she cares for her clients and she strives to maintain the attitudinal
values of the person-centred approach, seeking to form and maintain a relationship with the person, Dan, who has reached a point in his life where he realises he
needs not only to address his drug use, but also recognises that he has underlying
issues that need attention. He has taken a courageous step, coming into counselling, and Jeannie, his counsellor, appreciates this.

CHAPTER 1

A new beginning

Session 1

Jeannie waited for her new client to arrive. She has been working as a volunteer counsellor now for some 12 months. She had qualified a couple of years previously but had wanted to get some experience of working with people using drugs, or who had used drugs. It had seemed such a growing problem to her and she felt sure that the experience would help her in her future career.

It had been a challenging setting for her to develop her practice. She gave three sessions a week. The local drug team were glad of it; they were strapped for cash! She felt part of the team and she had gained a lot of insight. She realised how much she had changed since beginning. At first she had felt really wary of the client group. Drug users. She hadn't truly appreciated what she really felt about them. But as she listened to their stories and their struggles to get clean, or just get some control back in their lives, she had realised that she thought of them less and less as drug users, or addicts as the media loved to call them, and more as people, like herself, who happened to have made different choices in life in response to sometimes different, and sometimes similar, experiences.

Her new client was Daniel, 29 years of age. His keyworker in the team, Marie, had been seeing him for some while and had helped him bring his heroin use under control. He was now on a prescription for methadone and was slowly reducing that with her help, support and encouragement. But she had felt, and he had agreed, that he needed something more therapeutic. Marie had a nursing background and she knew that while she could offer him 'motivational interviewing', advice and support related specifically to maintaining his methadone use and relapse prevention, true therapeutic counselling was not something she was trained for. So she was glad that Jeannie was part of the team. She had referred clients to her before and they had generally appreciated her input, though one had only attended the once, finding it wasn't what he wanted, and another had needed encouragement to continue as he found it hard to organise himself to get there each week.

Offering an independent counselling service within the agency has many advantages. It means that the client has a place to talk through and explore their experiences in a therapeutic relationship with someone who does not have other responsibilities linked specifically to monitoring the client's substance use or liaison with other services. Having a clearly boundaried relationship in which the client is free to explore themselves in an atmosphere of warm acceptance and genuineness, where they feel listened to and can experience a sense of safety, where there is no hidden, or not-so-hidden, agenda concerned with their 'treatment', offers real scope for growth and development.

Well, Jeannie thought, drug users can be busy people, particularly those using heavily or using expensive substances. It can be a full day of robbing to maintain a heavy habit. Then getting to the dealer, going somewhere to score and then back round the cycle once again. She glanced at the clock and wandered out towards the waiting area to see if her client had arrived yet. He hadn't. She chatted for a while with the receptionist before returning to her room. She decided to sit and reflect for a short while before accepting that perhaps Daniel wasn't going to make it. After another ten minutes she went back to the waiting area to confirm that he had not arrived. Still no sign or word from him. Jeannie decided to make herself a drink. Was it coincidence that since working in the agency she had started to drink fruit tea? She had used to be such a coffee drinker but somehow she was aware that she was losing interest in anything that affected her mood – tea, coffee, she didn't drink as much as she used to, and ... She heard the phone ring in the room she used for counselling. It was the receptionist. Her client had arrived. She went out to find him.

'Hi, Daniel isn't it?' She saw a young man in jeans and a tee shirt on his own in the waiting room and he got up slowly as he heard his name.

'Yeah. That's me. Sorry I'm a bit late but, you know, had a few problems like, yeah?'

'Yeah. Come on through.'

Jeannie led him to her room and let him choose a seat. He went for the one by the window, leaving her the seat nearest the door.

'So, I'm Jeannie, I'm a volunteer counsellor here, though I am qualified.' She was aware that Daniel was looking out of the window, and didn't seem to be taking much interest. 'Ever had counselling before?'

'No, but Marie thought it would be a good idea, you know? Not sure what to talk about though.'

'Well, I want to begin by saying something about confidentiality. We are a confidential service and by that I mean that we do not pass any information on about you or anything that you have said unless you have given us permission. You'll no doubt be aware of all of this anyway, but what I want to say is that in counselling I won't be passing anything on to your keyworker, OK, unless you indicate that you plan to put yourself or others at risk, particularly children.'

'Yeah, I know, Marie has told me that. I'm not planning on anything stupid like that, and, children, shit, I couldn't hurt a child. Been there, I know what it's like.' Daniel was continuing to stare out of the window.

Jeannie was very aware of how Daniel had spoken, the words had sounded full of pain, and yet his face had remained expressionless and had not moved. 'You know what it's like, yeah, been there?'

'Yeah.' Daniel lapsed into silence. He was thinking back to the past, to some of the things that had happened. Nothing specific, although he knew that Billy's death was still with him and had got worse since he'd stopped using the gear [heroin]. But he didn't want to get into that now. He hadn't talked much about that to Marie; he certainly didn't feel he wanted to say anything to the woman sitting opposite him. He found himself wondering what she knew about drug use. She didn't look like an ex-drug user. Probably another do-gooder. Well, he'd give her a chance and see what happened. He knew he wasn't feeling so good and hadn't been for a few weeks now, but he really didn't know what to say. So he said nothing and waited.

'Hard to talk about?' Jeannie sat and was aware of wondering exactly what Daniel really wanted from counselling. She decided to voice it. 'What do you feel you want from counselling, Daniel?'

Daniel blew air out through his nose and raised his head slightly. Daniel. What his mother called him. Shit, he hated being called that. 'Rather you called me Dan.'

'OK, Dan, so I guess I'm really not sure what you want to use counselling for, but I see myself as being here to listen to whatever you want to say, to hear anything you feel able to tell me.' As she said these words she could hear Carl Rogers in her head in one of his demonstration video sessions saying something similar. She held back the smile. Her words were her own, and they were genuinely felt.

Daniel heard her words and there was something that sounded really genuine about them. He turned and looked at Jeannie, who was sitting looking at him. It seemed crazy but he really felt that she wanted to listen to him, that she really wanted to hear what he had to say. But no, no one wanted to listen to him, he was nothing, someone society despised and spat on. And yet he felt warm, strangely warm. And he felt his sense of desperation. It really hadn't been easy these past few weeks. He hadn't said much to anyone, didn't know what to say, but it hadn't been easy. He so wanted to get clean, to get off that damned methadone. But he knew he should be grateful; it had helped him off the gear. But there were times when he craved that beautiful buzz, of drifting into that place of forgetting inside himself. The methadone didn't take him there, well, not in the same way. Kind of dulled him but didn't give him what he really wanted. Fucking stuff, he thought to himself. He pulled himself out of his thoughts and took a deep breath, blinked his eyes and spoke. 'Sorry, miles away for a moment. I just feel,' Dan shook his head, 'I just feel so desperate, you know, I mean, God I miss the gear and I know I can't go back to it but shit, there are times when I so need it. Shit. Sorry.'

'No need to feel sorry on my account, say it as it is. Shit, there are times when you need the gear, yeah, and you desperately don't want to go back to it.'

'Can't go back.' He shook his head. 'My girlfriend doesn't use, she doesn't under-stand. Family, well, don't have much contact with them any more. See my younger brother sometimes in town but he's usually pissed. Don't have much to do with him. I feel so alone with it sometimes, you know?'

'Hard for me to know how it really is for you, Dan, but I do hear how desperate and how alone you feel with it.'

Dan nodded. Yeah, she's got it all right. Lonely and desperate. 'They've stabilised my methadone at the moment, said I couldn't reduce any more just yet. It's like it doesn't really hold me any more, except it does, I mean, I'm not clucking [withdrawal reactions] or anything like that, you know, but, well, it's feelings, I mean, I never really did feelings I suppose, always used something to take 'em away. I just feel so fucking awful sometimes.' Dan put his left hand up to his face and rubbed his forehead and through his hair, which was left standing up. He breathed in and sighed.

'So fucking awful, always used something to take the feelings away, but now . . .' Jeannie let the sentence trail off, having empathised with what she felt Dan was telling her and wanting to encourage him to say a little more if he wanted or felt able to.

'Does my head in all this.' He shook his head.

'What you are feeling, being here?'

'Yeah. Thought counselling would make me feel better.'

'Sometimes it does, but sometimes before we can feel better we have to learn to feel.'

Jeannie answers Dan's question but also places it in the context of what he had said a short while before.

'Don't think I really know what feelings are, you know? Crazy. Twenty-nine years old and not knowing what feelings are. At least, I mean, I suppose I do, I mean I get angry and I get sad, you know, but that's about all.'

'Angry and sad.' Jeannie kept her response flat; it didn't feel right to lift her voice as she said it to turn it into a question. So she simply added, 'About?'

Dan shook his head. 'Hard to know where to begin on that one.' He felt a rush of something inside himself, a kind of urge to talk about himself, something he rarely, if ever, did. But it somehow felt safe in this room, safe to just talk. He heard himself speaking, which seemed strange, like he was saying things but not really thinking about what he was saying, yet he was saying them, it was his voice, and they were things he knew he wanted to say. 'Life's been shite. Here I am, what have I done with my life so far, ay? Fuck all. Sniffed it, smoked it, snorted it, banged it up anywhere I could find a vein. Done some fucking crazy things, you know? Fucking crazy. Can't remember many of them, but I know they happened. All gets a bit hazy, you know?'

Jeannie nodded. 'Fuck all with your life, done some crazy fucking things, yeah?'

'Yeah.'

Silence.

Jeannie is matching Dan's language. If she was doing this just to sound as though she was in touch with him, it would be inauthentic and would probably leave Dan feeling that she wasn't being real with him, that it was patronising. But Jeannie is comfortable with the language, she does not feel uncomfortable with what she is saying and her words are owned by her even though they are empathic responses to what Dan is saying. Genuine empathy has to also have a ring of authenticity, or else it is the hollow, reflective parroting that gives counselling a bad name and leaves everyone thinking they can do it. Don't patronise a client by trying to be like them. Own your own way of being. But strive to be self-aware enough to know why you use the language that you do. Be authentic. Tell the client what you hear the client telling you, maybe in their words, but maybe in your own. The words are important but the tone of delivery is at least as important and often more so.

Jeannie was aware that although Dan was just staring into space, somewhere between herself and the window, she didn't have a sense that he was just blanking out. But she wasn't sure. She felt moved to voice her curiosity although she was also mindful of not wanting to cut across anything he might be experiencing.

'Wondering what you're thinking about.'

Dan heard her question. 'Teenage stuff. It all started out OK, I didn't seem to get into trouble, well, not to start with, but I guess it was getting on to the smack that did it. Bloody smackhead, that was me.'

Smack, or heroin, also referred to as gear, H, horse, brown, skag, junk. Comes as a kind of off-white browny powder. Usually bought in small wraps or packets of paper. It tends to sedate people and take them away from the reality of their world. Can be smoked or injected, sometimes sniffed. It leaves people wanting more to feel good, to regain the sensations and the mood shift. Powerfully addictive. Risk of overdose as strength of heroin can vary on the streets. Often it is 'cut' or mixed with other substances to make it go further, the user not really knowing what they are using. Users can die from overdosing. Injecting, particularly where needles are shared, can lead to infections and the spread of blood-borne diseases: HIV, hepatitis.

'Got me robbing, you know, had to keep me habit up. And a bit of dealing. Lived in this ... lived! Fucking stupid word to use. Fucking doss house, people coming and going all the fucking time. More like a fucking squat, over in town. Drugs everywhere. Shoot up, just stare at the wall. Don't remember much of it now. Got busted a few times for robbing, you know, shoplifting, cars, anything really. If it wasn't nailed down we'd fucking lift it. Shit we got through some stuff, you know? Fucking nightmare.' He put his head in his hands, looked over his fingertips and blew out a long, slow breath. 'Fucking nightmare.'

Jeannie nodded. She was very aware that what Dan was describing was outside of her experience, but she also felt a real curiosity as to exactly what it had been like to Dan. She didn't want to let her curiosity direct him though, but she did feel she needed to say something to clarify her situation. 'I've not been there, Dan, not had that experience, and I hear you describe it as a fucking nightmare and I'm really curious what you really mean by that? And I don't want my curiosity to get in the way of what you feel you want to say.'

Dan shook his head. 'You wouldn't want to know. Crazy times and I want to forget them, but I can't, you know, and the longer I seem on the meth, well, I kind of keep drifting back to those times. But I can't keep doing that, you know, I mean, I'm trying to move on, I want to move on, get my life together.'

Jeannie nodded and recognised that Dan was clearly not going to respond to her curiosity, that he was shifting his focus on to his sensed need to move on. She empathised with this, focusing on the last thing he had said, which it seemed to her he had progressed to and may now want to progress from. 'I hear that really clearly, you want to move on, to get your life together.'

As Dan heard Jeannie say this, part of himself felt really good, almost excited by it, but another part felt very scared at the idea. 'Yeah, I want to move on, but . . . shit, it ain't easy, you know?'

Jeannie was beginning to recognise that every time Dan said 'you know?' he wasn't necessarily expecting a response to a question, that it was his turn of phrase. 'You want to move on but it isn't easy.'

'No.' Dan looked lost as he said it, his face reflecting his desperation. Jeannie noticed it and responded.

'Fucking difficult, yeah?'

'Yeah.'

They lapsed into silence and Jeannie did not interrupt. It didn't feel awkward, rather it felt as though they had reached a common recognition that moving on wasn't going to be easy, and perhaps Dan simply needed time to be with this.

The silence is trusted as part of Dan's process. Jeannie maintains her attention and attitude of warm acceptance, but does not interrupt. It is a core feature of person-centred working that the client's process of being is allowed to flow wherever it needs to go. The client knows what they want to say, or not say, what is present for them and holds their focus. What the client so often needs is a sense that it is OK for them to be with whatever is present, that they will not be judged but will be accepted for who they are.

Dan was aware once again that it somehow felt OK to be with Jeannie, but he didn't know why. It was odd to sit in silence somehow, and yet it felt OK as well. He couldn't really make sense of it. Gradually, he felt a discomfort creeping over him and a kind of awkwardness that left him uncertain. He felt he needed to say something but he wasn't sure what. There was so much that he could say, but he wasn't sure where to begin, and he was aware that time had been passing and there wasn't too much of the session left.

Jeannie sensed Dan's unease. His facial expression had changed, looking a little strained. She decided that while Dan may not be communicating verbally, his body was telling her something. She decided to respond to it.

Responding to body language can be extremely powerful. Often facial expression can communicate what has not been put into words. It can reveal feelings that the client may otherwise be concealing or simply find themselves unable to put into words. Responding to facial expression should not include assumptions, but simply observations.

'Your expression has changed – seems to be a little strained.'

Dan tightened his lips and nodded. 'Yeah.' He took a deep breath. 'There is so much I could talk about but, well, I'm aware of the time and I don't know where to begin. Part of me wants to move on but the memories, you know, they can be so real sometimes.' He shook his head. 'Yeah, there have been crazy times, but good times too, you know? It feels like I'm leaving them behind and, well, trying to leave behind them for ever.' His voice trailed off as he said those last few words.

Jeannie sensed that Dan was moving inside himself as he spoke and, rather than stop him with a lengthy empathic reflection of all that he had said, simply reflected back the last two words which had somehow hung in the air. 'For ever.'

Conveying empathy is not simply about repeating all that a client has said. The context, the way it has been spoken and the sense of movement within the client must also be taken on board. Here the client has said a number of things, but the way he has ended what he has had to say has clearly carried a lot of feeling. Jeannie's response simply conveys back to him her appreciation of where he has arrived in himself. By responding just to this she is not directing him back but holding him where he is, and allowing him the freedom to continue as he chooses.

'Hearing you say that makes it sound like a long, long time.'

Dan smiled and blew air out through his nose, shaking his head almost imperceptibly. 'I loved my drugs, you know, they gave me experiences that I don't think I'll ever repeat, and that feels sad, you know. I mean, yeah, I really loved my drugs. Taken me on some trips, you know. Real crazy places. But the feelings in my head and in my body, nothing, nothing can replace them.' He shook his head. 'No, I know I have to move on, but . . . ' He looked into Jeannie's eyes. 'Can you really understand what I am saying?'

Jeannie felt herself smile. She knew that she hadn't used drugs, well, not like Dan had. Occasional spliff at university, but that was a few years back now. She liked a drink or two, liked that floaty sensation, but it hadn't become a habit.

She sensed the significance of Dan's question and she knew the importance of being authentic in her response.

Sometimes when a client asks a question, what is really being asked is for an opportunity to explore the need to ask the question; at other times the client simply wants an answer. The person-centred counsellor seeks to be empathic to her sense of what her client is asking for. If in doubt, this uncertainty can be conveyed to the client, allowing them the opportunity to clarify the directions they wish to take.

'I can really hear how much your drugs meant to you, though I have not experienced what I sense you have experienced over the years.' Jeannie noted the temptation to continue but realised that she would simply end up trying to justify herself as a counsellor working with drug users. She smiled inwardly to herself, remembering how she had fallen into that trap a number of times when she had first started working as a counsellor for the agency. It had been her supervisor who had drawn her attention to what she was doing. Now she felt much more secure in herself, realising that she may not have experienced the drugs or the sensations from their use, but she did experience feelings, emotions, and these were common to everyone, whether a drug user or not. She therefore added, 'Gave you lots of feelings and sensations over the years, yeah?'

'Yeah, powerful, really made me feel, you know, made me feel ...' Dan realised that actually he wasn't sure what they had made him feel. In fact, as he thought about it he realised that more than anything else they had stopped him feeling; well, some of them had anyway, the heroin in particular. Yeah, great rush but was it really a feeling?

'Made you feel?' Jeannie asked in response.

'Just wondering whether they really made me feel or stopped me feeling. I mean, so many sensations, yeah there were feelings but, I don't know, somehow it all feels a blur. Good at the time, though, well, mostly anyway.'

'Mostly good, yeah?'

'Mostly. But there were some bad ones, you know, shit. Yeah, some bad ones. Never knew what you were buying, see, and sometimes, well sometimes fuck knows what I was shooting up. Didn't care, just didn't care. Just so long as I got my next fix. Those were bad times, dark times, really dark times.'

'Really dark times, didn't know what you were shooting up.'

'No.' Dan suddenly felt very sad, almost depressed, as he thought back to those days in the squat, out of it, passing the gear round. He remembered how cold it had been that really bad winter, couldn't remember what year. He shivered as he thought about it.

Jeannie noted the shiver and kept to a minimal response. 'Mhmmm,' nodding slightly as she responded.

Dan took a deep breath and brought his attention back to the present. 'It's just so easy to slide back into thinking about it all, you know, and I can't do that, I know I can't. What do you think? Will counselling help me?'

'I really can't say how it will affect you. But what I am sure about is that talking about things and being listened to and to not feel judged, to be with someone who is endeavouring to be genuine with you, and to accept you as Dan, whatever your past, present or future, usually helps.'

Dan nodded. 'It has felt good to talk to you, and yeah, you do listen. You don't seem to say much, but that's OK.'

Jeannie sensed they were moving towards an ending of the session and she needed to clarify a few things. She smiled. 'So, you want to come back next week, or in two weeks? The choice is yours.'

Frequency of contact can be negotiated. The person-centred counsellor will wish to be sensitive to the client's perceived needs.

'Yeah, I'd like to come back next week. How many sessions do you think I'll need?'

'As many as it takes. Depends on what you want to achieve. You choose your own pace.'

'I really do need to go for this. Things have to change. I haven't really talked much about my past, but there are things I want to talk about another time.'

Jeannie acknowledged this and they arranged a time the following week and agreed to continue with weekly contact for a while at least, and review it in six weeks or sooner if Dan felt he wasn't getting what he felt he needed. Dan's response had been that at the moment he didn't know what he needed, other than to get some things off his chest and to try and get his head together, and get off the methadone.

The session ended and Dan left. Jeannie sat back down and pondered the session. She liked to take a few minutes to be with her thoughts and feelings. She was aware of feeling that she had made a connection with Dan, that there was a rapport beginning to build. She realised that it took time to build a therapeutic relationship, and she acknowledged to herself that this really was a step into the unknown for Dan. She admired his courage and felt sorry she had not said this to him. She got herself a cup of water from the dispenser and returned to her desk to write up her notes. Yes, she felt good about that first session. Her intuitive sense was that Dan was somehow deeply troubled in some way, that he had a lot of drug use in his past and she wondered what else. Fruitless to speculate, she realised, let it go. Trust him, he'll tell you what he wants you to hear and what he needs to communicate.

The importance of trusting the client's process cannot be too strongly emphasised as a core feature of person-centred working. Too much speculation can leave the therapist with a head full of assumptions that can then obstruct accurate empathic listening. The client has revealed what he felt able to reveal in that first session. Hopefully, he has felt heard and warmly accepted. The therapist has sought to be congruent, offering the opportunity of authenticity and genuineness to be present within their relationship. Drugs can distort congruent experiencing (Bryant-Jefferies, 2001) and can leave people confused and out of touch with themselves. Where a person has been substance-affected from early teenage years through into adulthood, a lot of emotional development can be lost, or distorted, simply because the person is unable to accurately experience themselves or a full range of emotional responses to situations and events in their life. Feelings may simply not be experienced and can feel quite alien when they later merge into awareness.

Session 2

Dan arrived a few minutes late. They had been caught out again by the traffic, and he explained this to Jeannie.

'So, how do you want to use the time we have today?' Jeannie wanted to allow Dan to choose his own focus.

'I don't think I mentioned my girlfriend last week, and, well, it's been a bit difficult this week. I mean, she's really important to me, you know, and she's a big part of why I'm here and wanting to get my head straight. She doesn't use seriously. She says she tried some stuff in the past, but nothing too heavy, a few Es, bit of puff, but nothing more. Says she never touched smack or mushrooms or anything like that. Anyway, she doesn't use much now and is really together, you know. I was having a bad day and, well, I guess I gave her some shit and we argued and she walked out and I felt bad, real bad. I mean, I was close to using. Shit, it was scary, real scary.'

'So she left and you really came close to using.'

'Yeah. But she came back. She'd walked round the block. I dunno, seemed like her walking out like that really calmed me down. Took the fire out of me. Felt fucking horrible. But she came back and we talked and made peace, you know? God, she means so much to me.' Dan put his head in his hands and screwed up his eyes. It wasn't that he was going to cry, he didn't do tears, hadn't done for years, ever since . . . He pushed a memory aside and took a deep breath.

'She means a lot to you, big reason for why you are here, trying to move on.'

'Yeah. We've been together a couple of years now, not sure what she saw in me. I mean, I had begun to get myself together though I was still using off the streets, you know? But she must have seen something in me. Anyway, she persuaded me to come here and to get some treatment, said she hated what I had been doing to myself and really wanted me to make a fresh start. Funny, we met at the A and E up at the General Hospital. I'd fallen over and had to have my head stitched. She was up there with her little boy. He'd managed to stick something up his nose and it had got stuck. You read about it, don't you, but never known anyone who'd actually done it! Can't remember what it was now, but they got it out. Anyway, we'd got chatting and one thing led to another, you know, and now we're living together and really trying to make a go of it.'

Dan continued to talk about his relationship with Gemma, and how she had been a real encouragement to him. As he spoke about her Dan realised more and more how important she was for him, for him now and for his future. Yes, he thought to himself, he was so glad to have met her. 'I have to keep control, I have to, for her, for me, for the future, but sometimes it seems so difficult.' Dan stopped speaking. Images were coming into his mind, memories from his past, people, places, they seemed to crowd in on him, his head felt like it was spinning. 'Can I have some water, I feel a bit spaced out.'

'Sure.' Jeannie went and got him some from the dispenser.

'Thanks.'

'You looked a bit overwhelmed by something just then.'

'Yeah. So many memories, just so many memories, you know, from how it was before I met Gemma. I was injecting smack for quite a few years, don't know why anymore, it was what I did. Full time. When I wasn't in prison, but even then, well, you know what it's like inside.'

Jeannie had heard talk of prison life and drug availability, and she could have nodded, but she didn't know what Dan's experience had been, so she offered him an opportunity to describe it.

'I know what I've heard and I guess I'm wondering what it was like for you?'

'OK. Screws were a pain but you do what you have to do to survive. Made a few contacts, you know, got by. Yeah, got by.'

Jeannie nodded and waited for Dan to say more if he wanted to.

'Well, part of the risk, you know? Had to start thieving to pay for my habit. Never got done for dealing though, managed to avoid that. But thieving, stuff out of shops, cars, occasional mugging, anything really, guess I wasn't too good at it. Always seemed in trouble when I was out. But you do what you have to do. I got by. But, you know, the last ten years or so, no longer than that, just a blur. Using, robbing, using, robbing.' Dan smiled. 'I know it messed me up but part of me wants to smile. It was mad, crazy, but it felt good too. Didn't have any cares, just didn't care. Did what I had to do . . .'

'Seems to sum it up that, "did what you had to do".'

'Yeah. I got by. Not proud of everything I've done, but I had to survive.' Dan could remember incidents from his life, the time he'd broken into that house, grabbed some cash from a bag and had suddenly felt the 'munchies' [hunger]. So he had taken food out of the fridge, sat down and had a meal. Just did it, seemed the most reasonable thing in the world to do, he was hungry, there was food, he ate it. Then he had heard the car pull up in the drive. Only just got away with that one, he thought to himself.

Jeannie had noted that Dan had drifted back into his own world of thought and she sat and allowed him to continue. He looked up. 'Drifted off, there. You know, it wasn't all bad, I mean, I never really hurt anyone, not really. I mean,

I heard of things people did to each other but I never got caught up in that. Guess I was lucky. Yeah, guess I was lucky.' Dan's thoughts had turned to Mickie, what a character. Didn't give a damn about anything or anyone, all kinds of trouble, finally had to get out of the area fast, too many debts and the dealers were after him. Said he was going south but Dan hadn't heard anything more from him. Never knew what happened. He knew what happened if you crossed the dealers, hell, he'd ended up being one, in a small way. They didn't give you any leeway. Beat the shit out of you, or cut you up, whatever took their fancy. Brutal bastards, but he'd managed to keep clear of it.

'Drifted off again, must have lots of memories.'

'Hmmm? Oh yeah, sorry. Geez, really finding it hard to focus today. Don't know why. Kind of feel close to a lot of what happened, you know?' Dan felt himself slide back into his memories again, and found himself reliving the feeling he got from the smack. Wonderful buzzy kind of drowsiness just taking him over. Just making him drift in himself. 'Just thinking about the smack, how it affected me. Seems hard to accept I'll never do it again.' Dan paused again. 'Good times, bad times. Yeah, that wonderful feeling, drowsy, relaxed, but it never lasted and then if I hadn't got a stash somewhere I'd be out looking for more. God it was awful, you know, when you thought you weren't gonna find any. Stomach cramps, sickness, diarrhoea, anxiety, shit did I get that bad, and shaking. Sometimes I had to be helped with the needle, you know, but I had to have it, had to have it. By then, well, it was good because it eased the pain, you know, but it was never a real buzz again, not like it was at first.' Dan went silent again, his mind drifting back to the first time he'd smoked it.

Jeannie had listened carefully to what Dan had been saying. She had felt the passion in his voice, he had really loved his drugs, she felt, and she kind of wanted to say it but she knew it was also coming from what she had heard others say. So she simply empathised with what he had finished saying. 'Never got the buzz again like the first time.'

'No. And you know, I can still recall that feeling. It was beautiful, shit, it was beautiful. Been chasing that ever since and never found it again. Now I have to accept that I never will. Now I'm having to deal with the effect of that search.' Dan shook his head. 'Beautiful. If only ...'

'If only?'

'If only I could feel that again but without getting all caught up in all the shit that went with it, but I know I can't. It's a dream, a nice dream, but that's all, and I guess it doesn't help dreaming about it, you know?'

That first hit of heroin, smoked or injected, is often the best a person ever has. They spend the rest of their drug-using career chasing that experience but it is never quite the same, and eventually it is no longer a real pleasure, but just a desperate act to try and stave off the withdrawal symptoms: pain, cramps, nausea, anxiety, insomnia, shaking, diarrhoea and a craving that just demands that you use again, whatever the cost. You just have to have it.

'Dreams are nice but unhelpful, yeah?'

'Pretty much. Now I'm on the juice [methadone]. Bloody horrible stuff, doesn't really do anything for you, doesn't make me feel anything much, but I just have to keep having it. Shit, I want to cut back on it but it's so difficult, so difficult. So many things to think about and it all just does my head in. Find it hard to concentrate at work. Not that it takes a lot of thought in what I do, loading up the lorries at the warehouse, but I sometimes feel like I want to run away from it all and just lose myself again in that beautiful buzzy feeling. But I know I can't. Tend to do a bit more puff on bad days, haven't kicked that habit and don't plan to at the moment. Well, Gemma doesn't mind that, she uses it occasionally too, but only occasionally.'

Jeannie nodded and wondered whether the reason Dan was drifting so much was because he had used puff before the session. 'Used any today?'

'Puff', 'grass', 'marijuana', 'hash', 'dope', 'blow', 'spliff', 'weed', 'ganja' are some of the terms used for cannabis. Cannabis is smoked, it comes as a resin in small brown lumps and comes from the cannabis plant. To smoke, cannabis is made into a 'joint', rather like a cigarette, but it can also be smoked on its own in a special pipe, often referred to as a 'bong', or even cooked to be eaten. It brings on relaxed feelings and makes people more mellow and friendly. It can cause people to be amused, to giggle and talk a lot. But it can also leave people feeling panicky, bring on paranoid thoughts and leave people confused and at risk of accidents. Smoking it can cause bronchitis and lung cancer.

'Yeah, stressed at work, came home and lit up. Yeah, really needed to chill out. Felt good. Yeah, feeling good.'

'Leaves you feeling good and I guess that may be why you are drifting around a bit this evening?'

Dan nodded. 'Yeah. Guess I shouldn't have used it but ...' He shook his head. 'Fucking awful day.'

Jeannie didn't have a problem with Dan using before a session so long as they could have some kind of meaningful contact. This she regarded as including both interpersonal and intra-personal contact, the latter concerned with the client's own ability to have, however minimally, some meaningful contact with their own process of experiencing.

In the case of a drug-affected client, it will be a matter of judgement as to whether psychological contact has been, or is being, achieved. It is certainly important to check it out with a client. The therapist can describe their sense of disconnection and enquire as to the client's experiencing. It may not require a great deal of contact for it to be therapeutic. For some people who are using drugs, who perhaps have rarely been given time and attention, particularly where they were unable to obtain this in their formative years, the presence of another person seeking to stay with them can have enormous therapeutic value. The person-centred counsellor seeks to communicate warm acceptance of the client, of the personhood of the client. Being prepared to be with a drug-affected client (whether prescribed, legally purchased or illicit) communicates something to the client, and can challenge their 'conditions of worth'. Of course, if the drug use has rendered the person threatening and the counsellor is genuinely concerned about their safety, then they will want to draw attention to this and may negotiate an ending to the session.

Dan had drifted again. He was aware of Jeannie and he knew what he was saying and what she was saying, but he also felt kind of floaty, like he was there in the room but somehow not really very solid. Felt good. 'I reckon that spliff has really got to me, Jeannie, I feel like I'm really struggling to be here. But it feels good. Yeah. So what else can I tell you? Used just about everything in my time, you know. Started on the glue and aerosols and stuff, and the alcohol. Well, the alcohol first, no, tobacco, yeah, remember nicking cigarettes off my step-dad when I was about eight or nine, and we used to nip round the alleyway and smoke 'em. Took us a while to get used to it, but we persevered. And then the alcohol. The older lads used to have it, they'd give us some, and we'd nick that from home as well when we got the chance. Still like the effect of alcohol, good feeling. I like the really strong stuff but only use it occasionally now. Used to drink a lot more, well, did everything a lot more!' Dan stopped again. 'I need a pee.' He got up and swayed slightly as he went out and across the corridor to the loo.

Jeannie waited for him to return; he seemed to have been taking his time. Nearly five minutes had passed. She heard the flush go and a few seconds later Dan reappeared in the doorway. 'Feel better for that. Look, I don't feel so good and I think I need to head off home. I've just called Gemma to come and pick me up early. Sorry about this; it wasn't a good idea having that spliff. Yeah, bad decision that one. Sorry. I've wasted your time. I won't do it again; it really isn't helping me.'

Jeannie responded, acknowledging what Dan had concluded and agreeing with him that it would be better if he could attend free of the puff, but that she also appreciated his openness about it. She didn't feel in any way judgemental; it had happened and Dan was as he was in the session. They agreed to meet again the following week at the same time and Dan headed off, deciding he'd have a fag while he waited for Gemma to arrive. He was a bit angry with himself for having fucked up, but he also knew he was experiencing 'don't give a shit' feelings as well.

Jeannie returned to the counselling room after Dan left, aware of how abruptly the session had ended and in a way still feeling herself a little hazy. She had noticed how when Dan had drifted into his own world of memories he had actually looked slightly blurry. She was glad that he had made the decision to head off. Seemed as though he had taken responsibility and he did seem genuinely sorry. She had listened to him and let him know that she had heard this before arranging the next appointment the following week.

Points for discussion

- You learn that your new client is an ex-heroin user, now taking methadone. What are you feeling? What are your expectations? How might they interfere with your empathy?
- Consider the issue around use of language that arises in Session 1. What is your response to this?
- Did you feel that Jeannie worked effectively with the silences that emerged during Session 1?
- Do you feel Jeannie offered the core conditions, and was she in contact with her client in both sessions? What examples support your view?
- How would you have reacted when it became clear that Dan had smoked cannabis before a session? What if you were aware that the client was drug-affected at the start of the session?
- Dan ends the session. If he hadn't, would you as a counsellor have continued with it? What would have been your reasons for whatever decision you reached?
- What effect might your decision have had on Dan? How might he have internalised it?

Summary

Dan arrives late and is at first unsure about counselling. But he feels able to talk to Jeannie and feels she is listening to him. He tells her how much he wants to move on, but keeps drifting back into thinking about his past and his drugs which were so important to him. He agrees to continue to come for counselling. The next session Dan has smoked cannabis before arriving. He keeps drifting off in the session, generally back to his drug-using past. Eventually Dan realises he needs to end it and is angry with himself for having 'fucked up'. Jeannie is quite accepting of him.

CHAPTER 2

Painful memories and the struggle to identify feelings

Session 3

'I really am sorry about last week, and I got a real ear-bashing from Gemma as well. I shouldn't have come the way I was, but I really felt OK when I arrived. But I just got more and more out of it as the session went on. And I realise that it didn't help much.'

'I appreciate your apology and I guess you needed to have that spliff at the time, meeting one set of needs, but then it affected your need for counselling.'

'Yeah.'

Jeannie had decided before the session that she needed to check with Dan what he remembered from the previous session.

> When counselling someone who exhibits symptoms of being substance-affected, it can result in the client making disclosures that they are later unaware of. For reasons of transparency, it is worth checking with the client at the next session whether they remember what they had disclosed in the previous session.

Dan replied that he could remember the session, that he remembered talking about what the smack had meant to him. He said that he seemed to have taken a trip down memory lane.

Jeannie smiled at this. 'Quite a trip!'

'Yeah, had quite a few of those too! Acid, yeah, really colourful stuff.' Dan stopped and he began to frown.

> 'Acid', 'tabs', 'trips' are some of the names for LSD or lysergic acid diethylamide, derived from the fungus ergot. It comes in the form of small paper squares with a picture on them and is swallowed or sucked. It takes people

> on a 'trip': they can see unusual shapes, colours can be brighter and more intense, things change shape, everything can speed up or slow down, strange noises may be heard.

Jeannie noticed this but said nothing, allowing Dan the space to express whatever he was feeling if he wanted to. She maintained her eye contact.

'Funny,' Dan continued after about a minute of silence, 'only once I can remember having a really bad trip. Fuck that was scary, fucking terrifying. Don't know why, just that one time. I was screaming and shouting, all over the fucking place. Horrible, it was, dark, very dark, felt evil creeping over me and flashing black and red colours and blood, fucking massacre, bodies everywhere, the smell of death. And travelling at speed and everything kept changing shape and moving around me. And I was moving as well, big, small, heavy, light, shit everything just kept changing. Like I was on some kind of ghost train but much, much worse, everything moving and changing, and the speed I seemed to be travelling, yet I wasn't really, it was all in my head. Felt it would never end. I was in it for ages before it began to fade away. Fucking frightening. Must have been a bad mix of something, I don't know. Took me ages to get over that one. Shit, I scored for days after that trying to calm myself down, get away from what was in my head.' Dan put his head in his hands and rubbed them through his hair. 'Never want to go near that kind of experience again. Last time I used anything like that, must be about ten years ago now. No, kept away from the acid since then.'

'That bad trip really put you off.'

'Shit, it was scary. No, kept away from it then, wasn't good for me. I mean, yeah, I'd had good trips, but that bad one ended it for me. Still used mushies though.'

> 'Mushies', 'happies', 'sillies' and 'shrooms' all refer to magic mushrooms. They are brown, dried-up-looking mushrooms and are usually eaten but can be made into a kind of tea-like drink. They give people trips as well and tend to make people laugh a lot, but users have to be careful as they can look like other mushrooms that are poisonous. They can also cause stomach ache, drowsiness and confusion.

'Mhmmm. So, the bad trip stopped your acid use, but not the mushies?'

'They weren't so intense. Kind of felt safer with them somehow. Didn't use them that often, but had a mate who could get them occasionally. Used to go round his place. Wonder what he's up to now? Lost contact. Lost contact with so many people over the years. Some moved on, some are dead now.' Dan shook his head. 'Yeah, a lot are dead now. Really sad. Lost some really good mates, you know? But it never stopped any of us. I mean, you know, it was always going to happen to someone else, never to you. Never to me.'

Jeannie nodded. 'Always to someone else . . .'

'Yeah,' Dan replied, before Jeannie could finish her sentence. 'Yeah.' Dan could feel a kind of quietness descending upon him, and it wasn't a comfortable one. He could see the faces of the people who he had lost contact with, some of whom he knew had died, but many others he just didn't know about. He felt … he didn't know how he felt. He felt sad but somehow he also felt detached, like he was watching the faces as if they were on a cinema screen. He could remember their names, Ricki, Pete, Allie, Lisa, Mandy, Marty, Joe, and many more.

Jeannie sat with the silence. She sensed that Dan wasn't just sitting there, that something was happening for him and she wanted to respect his silence. She sat maintaining quality attention on Dan, seeking to maintain openness and sensitivity towards anything he might wish to communicate to her.

'Good people, crazy at times, yeah, but good people, all with their own reasons for using, for doing what they did. Many had a messed-up childhood, abused, battered, thrown out of school, thrown out of home. Not everyone, though. Nigel came from a really good family but couldn't cope with the abuse at school, started using and dropped out from university. Fell on to the railway line, never had a chance. Express train. Just bits of him, all chewed up. Must have been quick. Waiting to get a train and he just stumbled, probably out of it, he usually was. Couldn't have known what hit him.'

'Sounds really vivid, Dan.'

'Yeah. It was. Can still see it, can hear the train and see him falling, and then nothing. The train pulled up eventually. Don't know what they found of him really, but shit he went under the wheels, just chopped up.' Dan closed his eyes. He felt awful inside, didn't know what to call it, but it just felt awful. He wanted to get away from it but he felt somehow stuck with it, unable to move his attention. 'He was a great guy, you know, could have had so much, but he was sexually abused, buggered up literally, couldn't live with it. Maybe he jumped. Looked like a stagger, he hadn't said anything. Maybe it was all in the moment, I don't know. Great guy, really sensitive, really cared. Cried whenever he heard about children being hurt. Guess he felt it so much from his own experience.' Dan sighed and looked into Jeannie's eyes. He felt as though he was searching for something but he didn't know what.

Jeannie held his eye contact, and sensed that something deep was occurring between them. Some part of Dan was reaching out to her and she had only herself to respond with. She felt her lips tighten. She had no words to say. She felt somehow suddenly very small and it seemed as though the perspective in the room had changed. Dan seemed somehow further away and yet he also felt so close, so very close. She still had no words and she sat with the experience, maintaining her eye contact, allowing the moment of connection to be. She had experienced this before and knew that it often signified a deep connection with a client when there was some kind of meeting that transcended in some way their individual identities.

Dan sighed again; he too had felt a closeness and a kind of warmth in that moment. It had felt like time had stood still, bit like a feeling he could remember from his past except that this hadn't involved a substance. He couldn't explain what he was feeling; he couldn't really distinguish his feelings. In fact, he wasn't really feeling himself at all, not in the usual sense. But he was feeling very present, extremely present. He took a deep breath and that seemed to change things. He smiled. Though nothing had been said he knew he had been heard, he felt heard, he felt ... he felt ... he couldn't find the words to describe it to himself. But he knew it felt good and somehow he seemed sort of more whole, though he wasn't sure what he meant by that.

He breathed in again and blew out a deep breath. 'I feel like I don't want to say anything, but I do.' The words came out almost as a whisper.

Jeannie nodded. She didn't want to say anything and take away the atmosphere that had been generated. She waited for Dan to say something more.

Dan suddenly felt a wave of emotion hit him; it came from nowhere and he realised he had begun to cry. Tears were running down his face. He didn't know why, but they were there, burning on his cheeks, making his collar wet against his neck. He could feel a lump in his throat and he swallowed, but it returned again, hot, burning. The tears continued. 'Sorry.'

'It's OK, it's OK.'

Dan had closed his eyes and put his head in his hands. He felt a sudden sadness, deep, deep inside of himself. 'So many people, so many friends, dead or gone. So many ...' He shook his head, slowly drawing his hands down to his mouth. He looked over his fingertips to Jeannie. He could see that she too had tears in her eyes. It felt good somehow to see them there; they somehow validated his own feelings, his own sadness, his own tears. He felt the emotion well up again. Jeannie sat feeling profoundly touched and affected by Dan, by what she sensed he was experiencing, and by her own sense of the loss that had become present in the midst of their relationship.

Dan felt the sadness begin to subside and he realised he was just staring at the desk lamp on the coffee table, just staring, no thoughts, blank. He sat. He stared. He did not move. He had nothing to say or to do, he could feel the blood in his cheeks and in the veins on his temple, and he realised he had tightened his jaw. He continued to sit. Nothing to say. Nothing more to say.

Jeannie said nothing, allowing the silence to be, the stillness to take hold of the moment. She respected Dan's choice not to move by not moving herself, seeking in this way to convey a body empathy for his stillness.

There was a sudden noise outside; a motorbike had passed by, accelerating up the hill. Dan slowly turned his head towards the window. He couldn't see the road but the sound had drawn his attention. He took a deep breath. 'I feel good for that, calmer, more at ease somehow. I can't explain it but it feels good, yeah, feels really good, and I'd like to just be with it for a little while longer.'

'That's OK.'

They continued to sit in silence for about ten minutes. Dan closed his eyes and just stayed with it; there was no longer the memories or the images in his head, and it felt such a relief. He suspected it couldn't last, but it was good to experience it. He became aware of a sudden urge to yawn, which he did, and it left him blinking. He scratched his head. 'Thanks.'

'Feels good?'

'Yeah. I need this place, here, and in myself. Yeah. Feels like I'm finding a new part of me, a part that can be calm and still, that doesn't have to be buzzing all the time.'

'A calm and still part of yourself, not buzzing.'

'No. And I am sure it won't last, but I want to enjoy it while I can.' Dan had glanced at the clock. Still 20 minutes or so of the session left.

Jeannie nodded. 'Enjoy it while you can, yeah.'

Silence again, but not for so long. 'I wish I could create this for myself, but it seemed to just happen and I don't know how. You know. I really wish I didn't have to take the juice. Feel it'll just fuck up what I've found. And I know I have to, but this has made me more determined to reduce. Yeah, I need to discuss this with Marie when I next see her, next week I think. But it won't last, will it?'

'I honestly don't know, Dan, I honestly don't know. But you are probably right.'

'It's like getting a glimpse of what is possible, how it can be, how I can be, but . . . and this may sound stupid, but I don't feel I've earned it? Does that make sense? Like it's been given to me but it isn't mine to have, not yet?'

'I think I understand. Like you've been shown something that you can have, but not yet. You have to earn it before it really becomes your own?'

'Yeah.'

Jeannie could feel herself smiling a little. 'Yeah. And I really hope you do earn it and make it yours, I really do.'

'Thanks. I appreciate that.'

They lapsed back into silence.

'I can't get over how different I can feel. I came in tonight stressed from the traffic. Gemma tried to get us through the traffic as quickly as possible but it really was solid out there. I was feeling stressed, then I felt sadness and now I'm feeling . . . I'm still struggling to know what I'm feeling.'

Jeannie had a thought as she heard Dan speaking. 'I guess it can be hard to know feelings.' Knowing how Dan had used substances over so many years, right through adolescence and throughout his adult life so far, she wondered how clear his experiencing of feelings had been.

People who use mood-altering substances during these formative years, when emotions and feelings are coming very much to the fore in the individual's experience of self, can find themselves in later life unable to distinguish feelings from each other. They can experience sensations which we know to be feelings but they run into each other, often leaving the person feeling profoundly uncomfortable and at risk of seeking ways of returning to their previously anaesthetised state. The emotional development can be constrained, leaving an adult with the confused feelings of a child. The counsellor working with the substance-using client, where there is a long history of use, will find it helpful to bear this in mind. It can have the effect of leaving the counsellor, who senses certain feelings to be present and being communicated, having what they sense denied by the client who simply does

> not appreciate what is being referred to. A client may need to develop their own emotional literacy in order for them to experience that the feelings they are experiencing and seeking to communicate are being received, heard and to some degree understood by the counsellor.

'Don't think I've ever really understood them, or maybe really experienced them. I think the moment a feeling emerged I would use something to push it away. When I was younger, much younger, I used a lot of dope. Liked the feeling. Don't know what it did to us but we used it after school. Helped me, I don't know, helped me feel better somehow, good in myself. And it was with my mates. We'd have a few laughs, silly things, fooling around. It all seemed wonderful somehow.' Dan could feel his reminiscence taking over. Yes, it had felt wonderful, and he missed those feelings, but what he had and was still experiencing now felt good as well. He felt kind of peaceful, unconcerned about things, feeling strangely able to cope with his life.

'All seemed wonderful?'

'Yeah, and I miss it, and what I am feeling now is good as well and it's not the same, in fact it is probably more real in that I haven't had to pump myself full of chemicals.' He smiled; there wasn't any thought to accompany it, he just smiled because that was how he felt. It was good not to have so much spinning in his head.

'Kind of an organic peace or something, sort of more real?'

'I like that, yeah, organic peace, natural. Yeah. Feels good. I need these kind of feelings but I guess I can't be selective. Just feels like the drugs have kept me blocked in and now stuff is rushing in at me and, well, I guess I'll find a way to handle it. Don't want to use again. It would just take me back. I know part of me likes to think about it, but I know that really, deep down, I do want to move on.'

The session continued with a further brief exploration of what Dan meant by moving on. He said that he wasn't sure but that it involved finding some peace, some stability, some normality in his life. Then they moved on to agreeing the next appointment and discussing the fact that Dan might have to work late some evenings and might need to change the day of his appointments occasionally. Jeannie was OK with this. There were only two nights during the week that she had regular commitments and the agency was open most evenings with staff cover.

Session 4

It was ten minutes into the session and Dan had begun by moaning about his day at work and how stressful it had been, how his supervisor seemed to have it in for him. He felt glad to have got that off his chest. He knew that Gemma was a bit fed up with him unloading on her, and he had deliberately said nothing when he got home so he could bring it to the session. He knew as soon as he sat down that he had to say something, clear it out the way. Yes, I feel better, he thought to himself, and shifted the focus.

People may come to therapy for particular reasons but it is not unusual for time to be taken to deal with what is 'on the top', as it were. It could be a grumble about something, or feelings associated with some event from the day. But it generally needs to be aired so that the client can more easily access the material that they want to work on in the therapy. Of course, offering warm acceptance, empathic responding and authenticity during this preliminary clearing out, or checking in, process, is in reality therapeutic, so although the focus may not be on the specific topic that has brought the client to counselling, nevertheless a therapeutic experience is being offered. The person-centred counsellor will let the client talk about whatever is pressing for them, trusting them to know what they need to address in the here and now.

'You know, it lasted a couple of days, that good feeling from the last session. And then it went. Or rather I guess I forgot about it in the heat of the moment really. We were sitting in the car at the supermarket, just getting ready to back out of the parking slot, when this idiot calmly drives in next to us and goes straight into the side of the car. Couldn't believe it. Fucking nutter. Stove in the back door on the passenger's side. Said he just misjudged it. I called the police and he was breathalysed. They took him away, over the limit. Serves him bloody well right. So we are having to sort that out. Maniac, being like that. There were children around, you know, and he could have . . . doesn't bear thinking about. Hope they bloody well ban him for a few years.' Dan had tightened his jaw as he had been speaking and clenched his fists.

'You're looking bloody angry.'

'Too damn right. Idiot. And now we've got all the fucking hassle.'

Jeannie nodded, and was aware that Dan didn't seem to be driving and she wasn't sure why. Had he lost his licence, she wondered, and put the wonder aside. That was her curiosity, not anything to do with what Dan was experiencing and communicating to her.

'So, that was the end of the calm, never really got it back after that. I mean, I calmed down, and the car is in to be sorted, and the insurance companies are talking, though I don't trust them too much. Often feels like they agree among themselves how to avoid paying out. Bastards.'

'Don't trust them?'

'No. No, been caught before thinking I was covered for things and then they show you the small print. Should be a bloody law against small print, stop 'em conning us. Well, that's what I think anyway.' Dan was surprised just how wound up it had made him feel talking about it. 'Bloody winds me up.'

Jeannie felt an instant response and the words came out without her thinking about it. 'Like a coiled spring.'

'Yeah, a very tightly coiled one.' Dan took a deep breath. 'But I don't want to spend all the time talking about this. Bloody idiot in that car, now he's taken up some of my counselling time. I should send him the bill.' Dan smiled at that, it seemed to lighten it a little, and he noticed Jeannie smiling too. 'Can you send it to him?'

'You'd like that, wouldn't you?'

'I'd love to see his face, I really would. Not that I want to see it again, mind you. Anyway, dammit, he's doing it again.'

'He's doing it again?'

'Yeah, OK, it's me, I haven't cleared him away, have I? Well, I'm going to stop talking about it, yeah. At least I didn't use on it, or take more juice. Glad about that. Didn't actually enter my head, funnily enough. Sure it would have done in the past. Well, I know it would have done. Everything was a reason to use, you know, everything.' Dan shook his head.

'Everything, yeah, anything and everything.'

'Yeah.' Dan paused. 'I talked last week about starting the cannabis after school with my mates. There was this guy one of my mates knew, friend of his brother. Don't know if his brother knew, but he got it and, yeah, it felt good.'

'Mhmmm,' Jeannie responded.

Dan moves on probably because he has felt heard and does not feel a need in himself to explore this further. Jeannie respects this by allowing him to take his own direction.

'Yeah, felt good.' Dan went quiet. Memories were with him again, images that he got from time to time but which he pushed away. Sometimes they came at him at night, in a dream, and he would wake up sweating, feelings of nausea in his stomach and sometimes struggling to get his breath. He closed his eyes for a moment. He wasn't sure he wanted to go near what he was remembering. He hadn't talked about it and he wasn't sure. He knew how it made him feel and he didn't want to go there, he really didn't. And yet, Jeannie seemed to understand him, didn't seem to judge him. Oh shit, he thought, but I haven't told her anything like this. What if she doesn't want to hear it? How would I feel if I told her and was left with it, unheard, made to feel . . . He didn't continue his train of thought. Change the subject. What had he been talking about? Yes, the cannabis, with his mates.

'Yeah, I guess after the alcohol, cannabis was my first drug. Hell, I nearly said my first love then!'

'Maybe that too?'

Dan sat for a moment and thought about it. 'Shit, that sounds weird. I don't like to admit it but you know, I think it's true. Yeah, first love.'

Dan fell in love with the feeling cannabis gave him. Where early use or first use of a substance inspires such a powerful effect it may be an indicator of the context for the use as well. Asking people what their first experience of using something was like can help reveal something of their psychological state. Comments like 'made me feel normal' might indicate that the person was previously feeling different, maybe even experiencing a disturbing state of mind. Or it may be described as 'brought a sense of relief', the person perhaps carrying painful feelings that they needed relief from. For others, however, the experience of first contact with a particular substance may simply be powerful for no other reason than the chemical impact.

Dan continued. 'I loved that feeling, you know. Different with alcohol, or at least it was then. Seemed to always drink too much and get sick. Used to make up these mixtures from the spirit bottles at home sometimes, put a bit of everything in. Jesus it tasted fucking awful, felt it was burning a hole in us, but we drank it. But the dope was something else. Liked the feeling. Made a change from what I felt at home without it. Bloody arguments. My parents, God knows why they got together, always bloody arguing. Me and my brothers used to huddle upstairs together in our beds. Dad was a drinker, would go out most nights and come back late, sometimes with a mate. We were supposed to be asleep but we rarely were, or if we were we soon got woken up. He'd often wake my mum up to get in. Bloody nightmare. No time for us, except when he wanted to do something. But more and more the booze came first. As I got older I learned to stay away more and more. My brother, who was older, he went off and joined the army, mainly to just get away from home. Don't think that was what he wanted, but it got him away.'

From talking about something he loved, and feeling heard, Dan has moved to talking about what he hated, what had contributed to the good feelings or sensations standing out for him.

Jeannie nodded. 'Had to get away.'

Dan nodded silently. Jeannie noticed the tears welling up in his eyes. 'It killed him.'

Jeannie frowned and leant forward a little, tightening her lips and grimacing. She felt a sudden surge of pain inside herself. She had lost a brother too, an accident. She was aware that her focus had left Dan. He didn't seem to have noticed. 'He drank too much one evening apparently and something happened, don't suppose we'll ever know what. But somehow he was shot. At first they tried to say it was suicide but there were no prints on the gun. He wasn't wearing gloves and you don't shoot yourself and rub the prints off, do you?' Dan sat in silence again.

'No, you don't.' Jeannie felt no wish to push Dan into exploring anything specific. She felt he knew she was listening to him and being as present as she could be for him. She was OK with letting him stay with whatever he was experiencing without interruption from her.

'My parents were never the same. My father actually stopped drinking, started going to Alcoholics Anonymous and has been dry ever since. Don't know where he found the strength, but he did it. Jake was nineteen when it happened, I was sixteen, just left school, first job. And Tony, my younger brother, he was fourteen, really affected him too. He's married, lives in the area, but I never really see him much. He drinks a lot, mixes with different people, see. Never really went to pubs, had my own mates. Can see my father's face when I came home and he told me. Wasn't long after my sixteenth birthday. I can see him as I came in.' Dan sat shaking his head. 'He was only nineteen. My father's face was deathly white, I can still see his face.'

'Sixteen, he was nineteen. Your father's face.'

'Yeah. He lost three sons that day, you know, though we are now talking again. Tony has some contact I know, but we never really got on much. We were, are, very different. I was more like Jake I think, at least, I know I wanted to be like him. Always looked up to him somehow.' Dan stopped for a few moments; he seemed to Jeannie to be collecting his thoughts. He continued, 'But that was the trigger that got me smoking the smack. Didn't plan to, got offered it a couple of days after the funeral, down at the pub.' He shook his head again and looked up into Jeannie's eyes. 'Didn't think. Needed something to take away the pain.'

Tyler makes the point that 'the key to understanding heroin is to recognise that, for most of these compulsive users, it serves as an antidote to a wretched existence – lives that might be full of pain, might be too complicated to manage, or – conversely – empty of any meaning whatsoever. Heroin promises neutrality. It promises *nothing*' (1995, p.75).

She nodded in response. 'Yeah, anything to take away the pain.'

Dan sighed. 'It worked. What relief. Beautiful, but it couldn't bring my brother back. Jake's death destroyed my mother. She's never got over it. My father has been so good for her but she lost it, big time. Compulsively cleans the house all the time. Everything has to be organised. Everything has to be perfect. My father seems to accept it. I guess everyone has their own way. I became a smackhead.'

'Yeah, everyone finds their own way to deal with loss, with shock, and you made your choice as well.'

'Yeah. Guess I'm not surprised, I mean, I was heading that way. I guess it was only a matter of time really. Tobacco, aerosols and glue, alcohol, dope, smack, acid, mushies, quite a career really. Even after that bad trip I still used the mushies now and then, but lost interest in them I guess when I started on the charlie, but it didn't last long. Wasn't me, somehow. Don't know why. Guess I prefer the "downers" rather than the "uppers", you know?'

'Charlie', 'coke', 'white', 'snow' and 'C' all refer to cocaine, which is a white powder and can be sniffed up the nose or injected. It tends to make people feel really confident and full of energy, but it can also leave people feeling tense, uptight and in a panic state, leaves you wanting more. You feel tired and depressed as the effects wear off.

'The charlie as well, huh?' Jeannie simply responded to the last disclosure but her questioning tone invited a response. 'But you generally went for the downers.'

'Yeah, I've done most of them. Body like a bloody test tube, I reckon.' Dan's thoughts were still with his brother though. 'You know, losing Jake like that just tore a hole in me, but I kind of feel I'm only really beginning to feel it now. I mean, I think I just tranquillised it with all the downers I've used over the years. Never really was a great one for stimulants, not until more recently when I started snorting the coke. But downers were my scene, and now I'm just on the juice, and want to get off that as well. You know, I really don't know when I last felt drug-free, you know? I'm going back a long, long way.'

'So, drug-affected for a long, long time, and now having to think about a future that's drug-free.'

Jeannie might have included in her response reference to losing Jake having torn a hole in Dan. But she hasn't, maybe preferring to stay with where Dan has got to in his narrative, but it could be that with the death of her own brother she is avoiding this focus but being unaware that she is doing this.

   Person-centred counselling demands a high level of self-awareness and sensitivity to what the client is communicating. Dan will not have felt this reference to the impact on him of Jake's death as having been heard. He might try to repeat it if he really wants it heard, although he might not risk not being heard again. It might also be that at that particular moment it is not that important to him for Jeannie to hear it. However, the fact remains that he has said something very powerful and it has not been picked up by Jeannie's empathic sensitivity. And because she is unaware of this it will be difficult for her to explore this in supervision. It is an example of why tape recordings of sessions can be helpful.

'Yeah. I'll get there. Last session reassured me somehow; that experience gave me a sense of some kind of inner strength. I know I lost it in the week, but it's there, I know, I felt it, I have to find it again. I guess my dad found it. Haven't really talked to him about it though. Maybe I should? I don't know. He must have found something to change the way he did.' Dan stopped for a moment.

'I may not have this right, but it seems like you are wanting to find what you had last session and what you sense your father must have found, something deep and strong?' Jeannie knew she was introducing different words but she knew she wasn't completely clear how Dan was experiencing what he was describing.

'Yeah.' Dan dropped his voice. 'I want to do it, I want to do it for my brother, for Jake. You know, he never really got into drugs, though he did drink a lot when he was in the army. And he's dead while I'm alive having put so much crap into my body over the years. I hadn't appreciated the rubbish that they can mix into the smack to make it go further – brick dust, anything, even heard that they use blancmange powder. Christ, could have ended up with a fucking trifle inside me. But I seem to have come through it. Probably the good thing was that I chased for most of my heroin use, only got into injecting later and only for a couple of years. Still struggled to find veins sometimes, but don't think I've got any real damage. I've been checked out, the nurse looked at all my injecting sites, and had blood tests, part of assessing me when I came into the clinic, you know? Even showed me how to inject properly if I needed to. Wish I'd known that earlier, when I was still using. Might have been a bit less painful and less risky. Never hit an artery, thank God, but more by luck, you know. That sort of stuff needs to be told to people. Kids shoving needles in themselves, no idea. They're gonna do it, why not make sure they do it in a way that they do less damage to themselves?' Dan shook his head. 'I'm going on a bit but it gets to me. What does a kid of fourteen know about how to handle a needle? I don't think the government really wants to reduce harm, they just want to stop people using so they stop thieving, that's all they're interested in, protecting the rich, protecting property. Bloody capitalists. All the fucking same, politicians, protect what you've got.'

Dan knew he was winding up again. That's how it was these days. Didn't take much and he just got more and more angry or pissed off about something.

Jeannie nodded and empathised with her sense of the build up of anger. 'Angry, makes you fucking angry.'

'Fucking well does. Fucking well does. Shit, I don't like to think of kids shooting smack and stuff, you know, but they're gonna do it. If we really cared about them, really cared, we'd show 'em how to do it safely. I know it happens in some places, but it's not enough. Makes me angry, but it makes me sad too.'

Jeannie nodded. 'Angry and sad at the thought of the effects on kids.'

Dan nodded. 'Yeah. And another thing. Injectable scripts. You could smash the smack dealers tomorrow if all services prescribed injectables on daily pick-up. Take them all out, smash their business overnight. Must be cost-effective. Must be cheaper for the government to pay for injectable heroin than the cost of all the thieving that currently pays for smack on the streets.'

Jeannie nodded. She had a lot of sympathy for what Dan was saying. 'You're probably right, you're probably right.'

In his book, *Street Drugs*, Andrew Tyler writing in 1986 offers his personal view that 'the world community must move – and fast – towards decriminalising the market so that it can assert some kind of control. If people are going to use drugs they might as well use unadulterated products made to an

> approved standard. They should have access to balanced information about the pros and cons of what they are taking rather than not-very-well-camouflaged government warnings whose credibility is near zero' (pp.19–20).

'I know I am. I mean, decriminalising it would stop it from being underground and if it was prescribed in a controlled manner then people would be less harmed in so many ways and the dealers wouldn't be able to sell it, would they? I mean, I know there are other drugs out there and no doubt they'd focus more on them, but we'd knock out the smack problem. I know I'd have been in treatment sooner if I knew I could have been prescribed something to smoke or inject. Hell, it's a damn sight easier than spending your day robbing. Might have even had time to hold down a job instead of drifting about!' Dan paused. 'Naah, suddenly gone off that idea!' He smiled.

Jeannie raised an eyebrow.

'But you know what I mean.'

'Yes, I do. And I agree, there needs to be a real rethink on everything. And I really appreciate hearing your thoughts and feelings on all of this, Dan, I really do. And I wonder whether this is the focus you want to have this session, or if you want to move on to anything else. Up to you.'

Dan has made some commonsense suggestions regarding prescribing injectable, pharmaceutical heroin. However, the downside is that it could simply encourage more injecting and mean there is more available on the streets. It would not be practical for supervised injecting to be introduced, as one hit does not last long enough, unlike methadone which can be taken once a day for the whole day. For some, injectable heroin would not be an appropriate substitute as they would prefer the culture of taking risks with what they are injecting. Nevertheless, it is a strategy worthy of serious consideration. It would be cost-effective, reduce harm and potentially save a lot of lives.

Dan glanced up at the clock, just a few minutes left. 'No, I feel good for having got some of this off my chest. Feel I've said a lot today, all kinds of things.'

'Yes, started with work stress, the car ...'

'Fucking nutter,' Dan muttered to himself.

'... your parents, your father drinking, your brother, his death and the effect it had, drugs policy and how angry and sad it makes you, and your own use as well.'

Dan smiled. 'You really have been listening. That feels good. Yeah. You know, I do leave here feeling better, well, except for that session when I was stoned, though that was a better kind of feeling too in its own way.'

The session drew to a close with agreement on the next session.

Dan left feeling positive. He still had strong feelings in his system and he wasn't feeling the kind of peace he had after the last session, but he did feel good.

Somehow he felt more real, like he was a bit more aware of himself, of what was inside him. He knew that he still had things to say, but he wasn't ready yet. He knew he would still get the nightmares and that he would eventually have to talk about them, but not yet. He didn't want to rock the boat too much... No, he felt in control and that felt good. He suggested to Gemma they pick up a bottle of wine on the way home and a few cans. He felt like he wanted to celebrate ...

Jeannie was writing her notes, struck by the wide-ranging nature of the session. So much had been touched on. Yet somehow it felt as though there was something missing. They still hadn't really focused much on any relapse prevention work or general support, but then she also knew that counselling was more than this. No doubt Dan was getting that from Marie, his keyworker. What she could offer him was space just to say whatever he needed to say, and to experience being listened to, taken seriously, feel accepted without conditions and be with someone who didn't have an agenda. She found herself reflecting on what therapy was all about. What are we trying to achieve, she asked herself? Yes, constructive personality change was how it had been described, but how did she see it? Two words came to mind. *Authentic living.* Yes, she thought, I like that, that's what we are helping our clients, and ourselves, towards: authentic living.

Points for discussion

- As a counsellor, do you need to have lots of knowledge about drugs and their effects to listen effectively to someone reflecting on their drug-taking experiences?
- How appropriate did you feel was Jeannie's handling of the silences, and would you have felt comfortable with them?
- When a client has little emotional literacy, how might you need to adapt your empathy to ensure that the client feels understood? What challenges does it present to the counsellor?
- Loss is a factor that is often present for clients using substances. List the losses so far that Dan has experienced and consider the emotional and psychological impact on him.
- Assess the impact of Jeannie's empathy on Dan, and how it may have helped him to explore what was present for him.
- Would more widespread prescribing of injectable heroin be an effective strategy to reduce harm? Discuss the pros and cons, and imagine you have to make the policy decision.
- What does 'authentic living' mean to you?

Summary

Dan describes some of his past drug use and in a silence connects with feelings of sadness connected to many of his mates who also used and who had died over the years. He realises that he finds it hard to describe feelings. He also refers to the death of a friend who had been a target for sexual abuse as a child. In the next session Dan begins by unloading about his work and his boss, needing to clear this out of the way before addressing other issues. Then he gets angry about a car accident. He reflects again on his past drug use and also talks about his early family life, his father's drinking, his brother's death and how it contributed to his starting to use heroin. Dan also offers his own suggestions regarding drugs policy to break up the heroin-dealing on the streets.

CHAPTER 3

Supervision 1

'So, your new client at the agency, how's it going, and how are you experiencing the relationship with him?' Max asked. Jeannie smiled.

'It feels complex, a lot happening and difficult to know where to start. His name's Dan and he is on methadone, prescribed. But in the past he's used all kinds of things. He's mentioned alcohol and tobacco, aerosols and glue, heroin, acid, cannabis, cocaine.'

'Quite a career. Using on top?'

> This refers to when a client uses a substance or substances on top of what they are being prescribed.

'No, but has come close recently. When his girlfriend walked out after an argument. Shook him up a lot.'

'Mhmmm.'

'But how does it feel being with him? Well, it actually feels quite good, I mean, it feels positive, feels like he is motivated and that feels good. He has a keyworker who he seems to get on well with, at least I think he does, he hasn't mentioned problems and often clients do if they aren't happy. He hasn't grumbled about his script which he might have done if there were issues on that front. So I think he is OK with the treatment package.'

Max nodded. 'Any concerns?'

'Lot of issues and I think it is going to be longer-term work if he stays with it. Right at the start he seemed to drift off a bit and reflecting back I do wonder if he was concealing something. Didn't make a big impression at the time, but since then he has disclosed that there were problems at home related to his father's drinking and his brother got killed in the army.'

'Disruption and loss?'

'Yeah, and he seemed to get into using quite early. He's talked about it a little, kind of reminiscing, as clients sometimes do, to what it was like. He has said that it would be good to have the experiences without all the shit that went with it. The death of his brother seems a bit mysterious, some kind of accident, not a combat death. Hit his family hard and yet it triggered his father into eventually stopping drinking. He uses AA and remains sober. His mother doesn't seem to have ever come to terms with it. Seems really tragic.'

'Must have profoundly affected your client.'

'He indicated it was linked to his starting to use heroin. Began smoking, but ended up injecting. Seemed to really be into it heavily, needing to rob to pay for his habit, and living in squats. Now he wants to move on, get stable and move on.'

'Big step for him.'

Jeannie nodded. 'Yes, it is, and I think that he still has a lot of chaos in his head.'

'Can you say a little more?'

'Well, taking it hard when his girlfriend walked out for a while, caught between reminiscing and feeling he wants to get away from the past, what sounds like a lot of disruption in his childhood. Can't have been easy and he really hasn't experienced life without being substance-affected for years, well, since child-hood, you know, possibly even before ten. He's said he struggles with feelings, with doing them and knowing what they are. I think angry and sad are the only two he mentioned as doing.' Jeannie thought back to when Dan had said that and recognised a common trait that often was present in people who had used substances as he had.

'So there could be a lot of grief still bottled up for him, for his childhood, his brother.'

'Must be. I do feel for him. He somehow seems quite lonely in many ways as well. I really feel he is going to struggle keeping stable. You know what it is like. People come to counselling for so-called ''support'', and it's just not realis-tic. People get uncomfortable in counselling, they are faced with memories and feelings that can disturb them, and they end up at risk of using more of whatever substance they are using, or lapse back into using something else. I feel concerned that this will happen for Dan, but at least his girlfriend is supportive.'

Max nodded, but his only real sense of her was that she had at some point walked out. He voiced it. 'When she isn't walking out.'

'Hmmm. I think he needs her. She seems to be encouraging him and he really wants to make a go of it. He also mentioned wanting to get himself together for his brother, too. Jake was his name. I think it's great that he is motivated, but I wish he was doing it more for himself. Seems he is doing it for others some-how – his girlfriend and for his deceased brother.' Jeannie knew from experi-ence and her own reading that people often needed to want to do something for themselves in order to make lasting changes.

'Leaves you . . .?'

'Uneasy. I just feel that Dan is somehow more fragile than he appears. And I can't quite say exactly why, but as I was coming over here today I was thinking about him and, yeah, I am aware of feeling anxious.'

Max could see the unease on Jeannie's face and he knew her well enough to know that it was genuine. She really cared about her clients, and he knew that some-times she could become too centred in an agenda of 'making them better'. He was aware that the person-centred perspective did not have an agenda but rather simply wanted to create a climate of relationship within which the client

could feel safe enough to explore themselves and from this develop constructively under the influence of the actualising tendency.

'Anxious about fragility, or something else perhaps?'

Jeannie sat and thought about it. She could see Dan's face. 'Can't say what it is
exactly. I want to see him get through all of this.' But as she sat looking at his
face in her mind it started to change. It became her own dead brother's face.
She closed her eyes. 'Oh, no, of course. I realised it in the session and pushed
it away. I know I've mentioned it before, that I lost Nick in a car accident.
He wasn't as young as Dan's brother, but I felt a pain when he mentioned his
brother's death in the session, and I think it is the fact that he seemed to have
died from an accident that affected me most. It was a chaotic time at home.
I really was close to Nick. I put it aside, I know I lost Dan momentarily, but I
think I regained my focus.'

Max wanted to communicate appreciation of this. 'Good. And you were affected,
yeah, and you lost your empathic contact with the client.'

'Yes, I shifted into me and I know it was triggered by what Dan was saying, I knew
it was my stuff.'

Max nodded. 'Yeah.'

Jeannie thought for a moment. She shook her head slightly. 'One of the things I
really learned from Nick's death is how fragile life is, how life is uncertain and
how important it is to do what you want to do today and not assume too much
about the future. It was quite a shock at the time, but that's, what, ten years
ago now. But that sensitivity hasn't left me. I do approach each day as being
in a sense not exactly maybe my last, but with an air of appreciation. I know
how fast things can change.' Jeannie stopped for a minute; she could feel a train
of thought developing in her mind.

Max sat and waited. He could see Jeannie frown and he felt it inappropriate to
disrupt her process. She seemed to need time to be with her thoughts.

'I was just thinking that Dan really is at risk. He has so many feelings I am sure are
linked to his past, and in particular linked to losses of different kinds, but I don't
know that he has really engaged with them. So many of the substances he has
used are downers, although more recently it seems he got into cocaine. Not
sure how that really fits in yet, he hasn't said much about that. But I just feel
that he has a lot to face in himself, and I wonder if he's going to be able to cope
without lapsing back into using something.'

'That's a real concern, you really can see him lapsing?'

Jeannie nodded. 'Yeah, and it, I don't know, partly makes me feel that maybe this
isn't the right time for counselling, and another part of me wants to trust that
his own process will get him through all of this. But ...'

'But ...'

'Well, it's the whole thing about psychological process and how substances, chemicals, affect the, I mean, I do firmly believe that we each have an actualising
tendency and that it works through us and if we experience a warm, accepting
climate of relationship, feel heard and listened to and feel we are relating to
someone who is being authentic with us, that we will grow and find ways of
dealing with what arises within us. And yet ... I really can see Dan using on

top before he gets through all this and I guess I am concerned that it may get out of control.' Jeannie was aware as she was speaking that she wasn't totally at ease with how she had expressed herself. 'I want to trust his process, and I do, but I guess I am wanting a particular outcome.'

'Which is?'

'Dan getting stable, resolving his underlying issues, reducing his script and maybe eventually stopping and moving on to a more fulfilling lifestyle.'

'That's your goal?' Max knew he was being devil's advocate, that Jeannie wouldn't want to think of herself as having goals for her client, and yet . . .

Jeannie felt the reaction inside herself. I don't set goals, she thought, but shit, do I, and if I do, am I setting Dan up with 'conditions of worth'?

The term 'conditions of worth' applies to the conditioning that is frequently present in childhood, and at other times in life, when a person experiences that their worth is conditional on their doing something, or behaving, in a certain way. The person-centred counsellor seeks to offer unconditional positive regard to their clients, not wanting them to feel they have to behave a certain way, or achieve a particular goal, to satisfy someone else's needs. Jeannie is wondering if she is setting Dan goals in her own mind which may then be affecting what she says and how she is when she is with him.

'I have to watch that. I really have to watch that. I need to be open and accepting of how he is, and of whatever choices he makes here. I have to stay with him, don't I, stay in his world and not get caught up in my own, even if my anxieties are for him. I'm at risk of losing him, losing the empathic understanding. And I cannot do that, at least not if I am to remain effective in working with him.'

'Yes, so you recognise the need to stay with him and while you may notice reactions, put them aside.'

Jeannie nodded. 'Yes, and it was my knowing how fragile and uncertain life can be, I think it has drawn out a kind of protective attitude in me, but I hadn't noticed it before now. I really do want Dan to get through this, and I am at risk of getting in the way of his process. I am in danger of finding it hard to accept if he uses or things take a turn for the worse. I can't do that. I can't have an agenda. I must leave that to his keyworker. I can't protect him.' Jeannie paused. 'I can't protect him from what is present within him, from what lies unresolved.'

'No. But you can be a consistent presence, offering unconditional warmth and a willingness to listen to whatever he has to say, or how he needs to be with you.'

Jeannie grinned.

Max raised his eyebrows. 'So what's that about?'

'He had a spliff before one of the sessions and just found it so hard to hold his focus. I really was accepting of it and did suggest that another time he might try and avoid it, and he did realise it. Got an ear-bashing for it from his girl-friend! I think he's learned that one, at least for a while anyway.'

'Until the next time it happens at any rate!'

'Yeah. He ended up going off early. He knew he was struggling, and I let him go. That felt important, to let him make that choice. He was apologetic the next session.'

'So he is in a sense using on top, though not an opiate?'

'Yeah, and I am not sure how much. The other sessions he hasn't seemed affected. But I'm not there to work directly on the substance use, that is for his keyworker, but on the issues, although there is always a crossover. He really has enjoyed his drugs, apart from a bad trip that put him off acid.'

The conversation around Jeannie's work with Dan drew to a close with Jeannie aware that she had to watch herself from losing sight of the need to simply stay in contact with Dan, providing the empathic listening and responding that would encourage him to explore himself, and to ensure that if she did disclose her own thoughts and feelings they were a product of their relationship and not coming directly from her own experience. She acknowledged, though, that she remained perhaps not so much anxious, more apprehensive.

CHAPTER 4

Panic attack and using on top

Session 5

'So, how do you want to use the session today, Dan?' Jeannie had watched him coming in. He seemed thoughtful, although she knew that was her interpretation of his manner.

'Well, I'm still taking the same amount of the juice, haven't reduced further. Had a review with Marie since I last saw you and she asked me about my alcohol use. She usually does. But that week I'd had quite a lot. Kind of started after the last session with you. Felt I wanted to celebrate on the way home, and we got some wine and a few cans, and I just got into it and really didn't stop much. I didn't drink loads, and we had quite a lot together in the evenings, but Marie pointed out how it would make me feel probably quite depressed, given the mix with the juice. Yeah. I've felt sluggish, just finding every day kinda hard, you know, it's all an effort. Made silly mistakes at work and got moaned at by my boss. Bastard. But since talking to Marie I've eased back and feel a bit better for it, but . . . Just feels hard-going at the moment.'

Jeannie nodded. 'Mhmmm, started with an urge to celebrate but a few heavy drinking evenings left you struggling.'

Dan nodded. 'Always liked a drink, you know, never seen it as a problem, well, I don't think it is. I mean, nothing like my father, or Tony.' He paused. 'But I am going to get it back under control. It doesn't help, but I wanted to feel good when I left here last time, I mean, I felt good but wanted to feel better I guess.'

'So how you were feeling wasn't good enough, wanted to feel better?'

'Yeah.' Dan sighed. 'And I feel so tired at the moment as well. Not sleeping too good. Well, it's kind of got bad recently, too many thoughts, my head keeps racing. Kept waking up in the night and now my sleep feels really disturbed. Hard getting to sleep the last two nights. Hot, sweaty. I know the weather's quite warm at the moment but I'm really feeling the effects. I'm sure the alcohol last week didn't help. But I've always drunk, you know, always been in the background.'

'So alcohol has been around for you for a long time?'

'Way back, back to when I was around ten, or thereabouts. Crazy times. Just getting out of it, you know, just needing to get out of it. Too much in my head. No peace at home. Needed to get away.'

Jeannie noticed that the expression on Dan's face had changed. It seemed sad, somehow; he had tightened his lips and shaken his head slightly as he had been speaking.

'I kind of sense a lot of sadness when you talk about that time, of needing to get away from things at home.'

> It is worth noting that Jeannie has been twice told by Dan of too much in his head, of racing thoughts, but it has not been empathised with and as a result she has inadvertently directed him towards a focus on his alcohol use.

'Yeah. Just found alcohol helped, you know? Took the edge off things. Made me feel, I don't know, sort of relaxed.'

Jeannie nodded. 'Relaxed and away from things?'

'Yeah, though we couldn't afford alcohol. Main thing was glue and aerosols. They were cheap, well, actually, easy to nick. Yeah, used them a lot.' Dan took a deep breath and sighed. 'Used to go round this shop near where we lived and get them and go round to this sort of wasteland nearby – old warehouses and stuff. Yeah. Used to feel really weird, kinda drunk, spaced out, really high and, I dunno, we laughed a lot, fooled around, did things, you know, we mightn't have otherwise done. Messin' around.' Dan sighed again, slowly and heavily.

> Aerosols, lighter-gas tubes or tins of glue are generally sniffed or breathed in. It is dangerous to spray them into the mouth or nose; spraying gas this way can cause instant death. It is also dangerous to mix sniffing with drinking alcohol. The effect of sniffing and breathing these substances is that the user can feel dizzy. They can also feel sick, may be drowsy and lose control of their balance. Obviously, this can cause them to fall and this may lead to accidents. Sometimes the effect is enhanced by sniffing with a plastic bag over the head, but this is again highly dangerous. It makes breathing difficult and can lead to suffocation.

Jeannie sensed he was remembering his past experiences, yet while he was talking about messing around and laughing a lot, his body language and expression seemed really heavy. They didn't tie up. Jeannie responded to what Dan was communicating.

'Seems like you are talking about laughing and messing around but it seems very heavy somehow as well.'

Silence. After a while, Dan spoke again. 'Yeah.' He didn't say anything else. He just continued to sit, staring down at the floor. Jeannie had noticed that while he was still, he was picking at his fingers. Not harshly, but continuously. Jeannie respected that Dan was experiencing something within himself and she did not want to disturb that. She allowed the silence to continue. Dan continued to pick at his fingers, although he was completely unaware that he was doing it.

Minutes passed. 'I'm here if there is something you want to say, Dan.' Jeannie spoke softly, not wanting to draw Dan's attention out from wherever he was focused, but wanting to let him know she was there. Dan did not hear her. He was back in that warehouse again, a scene that had played over and over again in his mind down the years. Not constantly, but it came back in dreams. Some of the drugs, well all of them, had helped him push it away, but it kept coming back. Billy. Poor Billy. Dan closed his eyes and took a deep breath. He didn't want to talk about it. He didn't want to go back there again. But the scene was so clear. He couldn't push it aside. Yet he desperately wanted to. He felt scared, no, fear. No, it was worse than that. He could feel his heart pounding faster and he was aware that his breathing had become more rapid. He couldn't stop it. It seemed to get faster and faster. Coming rapidly, short and sharp breaths. He felt dizzy, his mouth was dry, his head was spinning. He tried to raise his head, but couldn't move it. His breathing continued in short, sharp breaths.

Jeannie had been watching Dan as he sat there and noticed his breathing suddenly changing. 'Dan, are you OK?' No response. 'Dan, can you raise your head?' Still no response.' His breathing had got faster still. 'Dan, I am going to hold your hands and I want you to try and take slightly larger breaths, try and slow your breathing down by taking slightly larger breaths.' She reached over and took his hands; they were cold and clammy.

Dan heard Jeannie and tried. His breathing became quite jagged as he struggled to breath in more fully without breathing out immediately. He could hear the sound of the breath in his throat. He was breathing though his mouth.

'Dan, try and close your mouth between breathing in and breathing out. And squeeze my hands.' She wanted to distract him a little from his breathing, to try and reduce some of the anxiety that was clearly driving what was happening to him.

'Huuhh. Huuhh. Huuhh.' Dan struggled to slow his breathing down.

'I'm going to open the window and let in some fresh, cooler air.' Jeannie got up and did so, and came back, taking Dan's hands again.

As the cool air reached his face, Dan felt himself breathe it in more deeply; it helped slow him down a little more. He gradually began to feel the dizziness fading. As he took another deep breath he found he could raise his head. His breath came out in little bursts. He breathed deeply again, slower, closed his mouth and held it for a moment before breathing out again. He swallowed, taking another breath, and blew this one out slowly.

'How are you feeling? Can I get you some water?'

'That was frightening. I thought I'd lost it. I've had attacks like that in the past, but that really did feel bad.' He had his eyes closed as he spoke. He opened them, looking across at Jeannie. 'Yes, some water would be good, thanks.' Jeannie went off to get some.

When she returned, Dan was sitting rubbing his eyes and yawning. 'There you go.'

'Thanks.' He drank it and put the cup down on the table. 'I've felt like that before at different times, but that was quite intense. I feel quite weak now, my arms feel kind of rubbery, you know.'

'You also look a bit tight, your shoulders?'

'Oh yeah.' He moved them around to free them off; he hadn't noticed how tense they had become. 'That's better.' He yawned again.

'You seemed to be really lost in thought before that happened.'

'Yeah, I was, thinking back to those early days, you know. Lots of memories.' Dan could feel anxiety rising inside himself again. He didn't want to go back there. He wanted to change the focus of the session. He yawned again. 'That really took it out of me.' He glanced up at the clock and yawned again. 'Oh dear, can't seem to stop now.' He paused and collected his thoughts together. 'So, I guess I feel I've got some ideas from talking it through with Marie about what to do about my drinking. The methadone feels stable at the moment. I just need to get myself together.'

Jeannie recognised that Dan wasn't focusing on what had just happened or about whatever he had been experiencing prior to the panic attack. Yet she wanted to respect his choice in this. If he didn't want to talk about something, that was his choice. She didn't want to push him; clearly something had disturbed him and she wanted him to feel safe to disclose it when the time was right for him.

A key element to person-centred counselling is staying with the client and trusting that they will communicate whatever they need the counsellor to hear. The counsellor trusts the client as knowing what is present for them that they wish to address. Sometimes, they feel ready to reveal something that is painful, but at other times, as in this example, the client feels, for whatever reason, that they do not wish to disclose something or reconnect with memories of past experiences. The person-centred counsellor trusts the client's process in this.

Yet Jeannie was also aware that what had just occurred had been quite dramatic and, in a sense, it was a form of communication. Dan's bodily reaction was communicating something related to whatever Dan had been thinking about, reliving, whatever it was that was in his mind at the time. She wondered whether to say something and decided to at least make visible her awareness of the choice of direction that Dan might want to take.

'Your body really did express some high anxiety back then, Dan, and I really want to acknowledge that, and I want to say that I also hear you saying about wanting to get yourself together.' As she said it Jeannie sensed that she needed to discuss her decision in supervision.

'I do want to get myself together.' He definitely did not want to go into his feelings about his memories. He could feel himself saying to himself that he was strong enough, he'd got through over the years, and he'd continue to do so now. 'I want to really make a go of things with Gemma, you know? She's so good for me.'

'Good for you?'

Dan smiled. 'She doesn't take the bullshit I try to give her.' He shook his head and smiled even more. 'I don't know, she seems to care about me and look after me.'

Jeannie felt herself experiencing a sense of Dan as a child needing looking after, of not being sure how to be an adult.

'That feels important for you, to be cared for and looked after.'

'Yeah, yeah, it is.' Dan spoke slowly. 'I never really felt that in the past, you see, never really felt cared for. She's good for me, though I know I don't always like it. Sometimes she says she feels like she has two children in the house.' Dan grinned, and as he did so he seemed to suddenly be much younger to Jeannie.

'You feel like a child?'

'Yeah, I do. She tells me I get in the way, get under her feet. Yeah, we have arguments, people do, don't they?'

'They do. So I am wondering whether the arguments make you feel like a child?'

'I kind of sulk when we argue, at least afterwards. She huffs and puffs about things and I suppose I get a bit moody. But she starts it, telling me off about something I've not done, or not done right. Sometimes I react, and sometimes I deny it, and sometimes I just go into another room and try and ignore it all.'

'So you have a range of reactions then, yeah?'

'Yeah, but I never really win. I usually end up doing what she wants. I don't seem to be able to really argue back. Seems I want to keep the peace, you know, not cause arguments. I don't like them. I feel, I don't know, just don't like them.'

'Don't like arguments with Gemma.'

'Not just Gemma. I just don't feel comfortable. Leaves me unsettled, on edge, just don't like it. Do anything to just settle everything back down again.'

Jeannie felt her thoughts drift to Dan's past, the arguments at home; he must have had so much of it and maybe now he wanted to avoid it.

'Anything to avoid an argument or settle it back down again?'

Dan nodded. His mind had gone back to huddling up with his brothers, hearing the arguments and the fights downstairs. He closed his eyes. 'I wish they would stop sometimes, but they just never seemed to. I mean, they must have done, it can't have always been arguments, but I don't remember. I just remember the arguments. I guess my memory's not too good either, there are big gaps. I think I've probably messed it up with all the gear. Don't find it easy to remember things even now.' He shook his head. 'Think I've messed myself up a bit. Feel bad about that. Looking back so much of it is hazy, and there are chunks missing, and then there are really sharp bits that are really clear.' He put his face into his hands. He took a deep breath, and then let it out. He didn't take another breath for a few moments, but stayed sitting with his elbows on his legs, his face in his hands. He gradually drew his hands down his face and slowly breathed in again. 'Drugs have messed me up, haven't they?'

'That how it feels? Messed up by the drugs?'

'Yeah. Yeah. And I'm still using, I mean, there's the juice but I'm drinking, I smoke puff regularly, I smoke cigarettes. I'm still full of chemicals, still full of fucking shit.' As he spoke his words got stronger and louder.

Jeannie empathised, matching his tone of voice as she spoke. 'Full of chemicals, full of shit, yeah? That's how it feels.'

'I've got to get free of all of this. I sometimes feel like bits of me are missing, like I'm not all here. Fuck knows where I am. I don't know. Sometimes I can feel really positive, but other times, like now, I can feel really depressed about it all. Seems like an endless struggle. And I'm still struggling. I need that script. Can't cope without it. There are days when I am so grateful for it, and other days when I am just so fucking frustrated by it all. I want to break free.' He snorted out a breath. ' "I want to break free." '

'Yes.' Jeannie was aware that Dan wanted to break free from his reliance on sub-stances, and she was aware of wondering what else. 'You want to break free.' She left her response as an empathic one and allowed the silence to be for Dan to have the opportunity to focus on this urge, this need, this drive that was pre-sent within himself. Some aspect of his nature wanted to break free and move on. Yet he still needed the chemicals, the drugs. He still needed to be affected by them.

'I mean, I am stable and that, but there are days when it is so fucking hard. I really feel I want to go out and get some gear again. And I know I can't. And I won't, but some days, it's just so fucking hard.'

'You want to and you can't, and it's so fucking hard not to.' Jeannie was aware of feeling affected by the tone and strength of what Dan was saying. She added, 'I'm really touched by your struggle.'

'It isn't easy. Just feel like there's no buzz any more, just existing. Go to work, get moaned at, go home, have a drink, get moaned at, go to bed, can't sleep, get up, go to work. Never ends. Too boring.'

'Just bored with it all.'

Dan knew he wasn't only bored; there were good times, but just at this moment he just felt fed up with it all. 'Endless. And I feel so tired.' Dan, as he spoke, was aware of how heavy-eyed he felt. His eyes seemed full of fine grit, hot and burn-ing under the eyelids, particularly at the bottom. Blinking didn't really seem to clear it. He yawned again. 'I'm drifting. I'm not really concentrating, Jeannie, I'm not really with it at the moment. That panic earlier has wiped me out. I just want to close my eyes, lie back in this chair and just relax.'

'OK, so just lie back and close your eyes. That's OK.'

Dan did just that. He felt so tired. He leaned back into the chair, closed his eyes and let out a long, slow breath. He didn't feel he was going to go to sleep, his eyes were heavy and he did feel tired, but he could feel so much going on inside himself as he sat there. He was very aware of the cool air in his nose and of that coolness touching the skin on other parts of his body. It wasn't uncomfortable, but it gave him a sense of his own edges, at least in places. But his hands felt heavy, and the fingers and palms seemed somehow slightly tingly. His arms were heavy, they just hung down, his hands resting on his thighs. Yet in his head his thoughts were spinning but he found himself somehow just watching them spin. It was like they were rushing around and he just couldn't be both-ered to do anything about them. He hadn't the energy. He stayed in the chair, his head back on to the top support which was fortunately padded and comfor-table. He took another deep breath and as he breathed out he could feel a slight churning sensation in his stomach. Kind of tickly but also uneasy. He took another deep breath and focused on that.

'It's no good, I think I'm going to have to head off. I just feel so tired. And I haven't had any puff this time, honest.'

'I believe you. Well, there's only about ten minutes or so of the session left. Do you want to sit quietly until Gemma arrives, or what?'

'Yeah. I really appreciate you giving me the time and the space for this. It feels good to just sit and be. My head's racing but somehow I don't care. Just want to sit and relax.'

Jeannie had an image come to mind. 'Like a big, floppy rag doll.'

Dan thought for a moment. 'No, actually more like a puppet who's had his strings cut.' With that he let his head roll from side to side. 'Oh. I can feel my neck creaking as I do that.' He stopped. He continued sitting. 'I feel really calm, but not like the other session, this is definitely a tired calm.' A minute or two more passed. 'OK, time to move on.' Dan opened his eyes, yawned again and slowly got to his feet. They confirmed the appointment for the following week and Dan headed outside for a smoke and to see if Gemma had arrived, which she had.

Session 6

It was now ten minutes after the session was due to start with Dan and there was no sign of him and there had been no message. She was aware that he had been late before and so she wasn't overly concerned. The last session had ended with Dan seemingly relaxed, although she had continued to be concerned about whatever it was that had triggered that panic attack. However, he had not wanted to discuss it. She respected that. Time was passing as Jeannie waited for Dan to arrive. There was no sign of him yet. She sat and reflected on the sessions they had had and how she felt about the therapeutic relationship she was building with Dan. It still felt like early days. He had told her a lot about his past and yet there were still gaps. She didn't have a really clear picture about his parents and his relationship with them, or his period in and out of prison. She was also aware that she didn't really know much about his cocaine use; however, she also recognised that it wasn't for her to know all these things. He had a keyworker, and she was there to offer therapeutic counselling. Enabling him to have a place to talk through issues that were confidential. Something, she had soon realised when she began this work, that was often a new experience to clients who had long ago learned to keep quiet about their inner worlds of thought and feeling.

Time continued to pass. She was aware that Dan had come into counselling at a time when he was relatively stable. He wasn't still using off the streets, living off his wits, robbing to maintain his habit. That's one good things about methadone; it does help some people get away from street use and from the perils of injecting. She also recognised, though, that the culture could be to take risks, that for some groups of users 'dirty hits' were part of the whole experience, often linked, she felt, to low self-esteem and a need to put one's health at risk. People injecting off the street often said they didn't care; they just wanted to run with the experience, and at times feel the thrill of not knowing quite what their gear was cut with – bit of brick dust maybe, chalk, whatever.

No, at least Dan seemed fairly stable and was really only starting out in counselling. She expected it to be a bit chaotic to begin with.

> Many injecting drug users have become conditioned into a chaotic lifestyle, normalising it either from much earlier in their lives or as a result of their use and the culture and lifestyle that developed around it. And yet within this chaos there was a need for order, the order that allowed them to get the money to buy their next stash, find the dealer, use and then begin the cycle again.

She wanted to help Dan experience himself in the therapeutic relationship. She knew it would be hard, that it would draw his natural defensiveness to the surface, that it would be uncomfortable for him at times to adapt to being offered unconditional positive regard by someone giving him time without an agenda on him or his life. She wanted to be there to hear what he wanted to say, to be touched by what he was feeling about his past, present, or hopes for the future. She trusted that within him, as in everyone, there was a tendency towards growth, towards development and the achievement of satisfaction from the choices made in life. So much of his experience of life had been chemically affected by drug use.

She reflected on the terrible challenge faced by society. So many young people and children were now becoming chemically affected in their development, and the longer-term effects were not really fully known. She was aware of her own concerns and anxieties, wondering what possible damage was being done to the brains and central nervous systems of young people that, long term, could have significant impact on their quality of life and ability to function to their fullest potential.

She noted a deep sadness inside herself, thinking of the scale of the problem and wondering what difference she could make. She sat staring at the wall for a minute or so, and then brought her thoughts back to Dan. No, she couldn't change society, but she could help the individuals that were referred to her to experience being warmly accepted as the person that they are. So they used drugs, but they were more than drug users, or 'addicts' as the press loved to call these human beings. She wanted to relate to them as individual people and help them to experience being related to as a unique person in their own right.

Jeannie was still very much centred in her thoughts when there was a knock on the door. She felt her body jump and she blinked and brought herself back into the room and the present.

'Yes?'

'Telephone call for you.'

'OK, I'll come and get it . . . Hello, Jeannie speaking. How can I help?'

'Oh hi,' the voice sounded breathless, 'I'm Gemma, Dan's girlfriend. Hmm. He's in hospital, at least I'm phoning from the hospital, not sure what's happening here. He got brought in a while ago and they are doing tests. So obviously he won't be with you. Sorry I couldn't call before but it was all very hectic. He, I don't know, he'd gone and started injecting and something happened. He passed out a while ago, feeling really weird, he said, and I dialled 999. I don't know any more at the moment. Oh God, I don't know what else to do, I mean, he looked awful and they really seemed concerned about him.'

'Thanks for letting me know, must be an awful shock and I'm sure they will sort out what has happened.' Jeannie deliberately avoided overly empathising; she didn't want to encourage Gemma to be with her feelings at this time. It wasn't appropriate. Gemma needed reassurance. 'Presumably they are checking him over at the moment?'

'Yes, and I'm waiting to hear what they have to say and what they are going to do.'

'Look, Gemma, I really appreciate you calling, and please let us know what's happening. When he's out let us know and we'll organise another appointment.' Jeannie wanted to be positive. She knew that, well, all kinds of things might have happened, and she didn't want to start interrogating Gemma. Dan was in the right hands at the moment, and Gemma needed support.

'Yes, I will. Look, I have to make some more calls. Thanks for listening.'

'That's OK. I'm sorry to hear what has happened and I'm sure that we'll help Dan make sense of it all and get back on track again. Do you want me to let his key-worker know?'

'Yes, can you? And if I know any more I'll get back to you.'

'OK. Take care. It'll be OK. Dan's where he needs to be. It'll be OK.'

'Yes, I'm sure you're right. I want . . . Silly fool, why did he go and do it? I know why, he said he'd dropped his methadone – why can't they put in plastic bottles? When I was away at the weekend. Oh well, look, must go. Thanks again.'

'Thank you for calling. We appreciate it and we'll all be sending Dan positive thoughts, you know?'

'Yeah. Thanks. Bye.'

'Bye.'

Jeannie heard the phone go click and she slowly put down the receiver. She hadn't expected that. The receptionist looked across. 'Bad news?'

'Yeah, client in hospital. Thanks for calling me to the phone.'

Jeannie walked back to the counselling room. Dammit, she thought, damn, damn, damn. He didn't need this. She took a few deep breaths and decided the first thing was to note down her conversation in the notes while it was fresh in her mind, and then leave a message for Marie, who would be in next day. Yes, she thought, why doesn't methadone get dispensed in plastic bottles? Would be a sensible harm-reduction strategy.

Jeannie was concerned rather than upset. She had warmed to Dan, and really appreciated the momentous struggle he was facing in his life, and the huge changes he was trying to make. She guessed he may have tried to cope without anything over the weekend but just couldn't cope. The agency isn't open 24 hours and he probably didn't think about going to his GP – not that every GP is happy to prescribe in these circumstances. Must have started to inject, probably had to continue till Gemma got back. And something has gone wrong. She put away the file, and went to get a drink. One of the other counsellors was around and she went to have a quick chat about it. She didn't feel any pressing need to trouble her supervisor, but just felt she needed to tell someone.

Many services will not issue another prescription in these circumstances, or where it is claimed a prescription has been lost, in order to minimise the risk of 'double-scripting'.

Points for discussion

- How would you have responded if Dan had been your client and had experienced a panic attack?
- Should Jeannie have been more proactive in keeping Dan focused on the cause of his panic attack? If so, how would this equate with person-centred working?
- Discuss the quality of Jeannie's presence as you sense it to be from reading Session 5.
- How do you explain the experience of tiredness that overwhelmed Dan?
- Jeannie speaks to Dan's girlfriend. Was this appropriate and, if so, why? In what situations would you not speak to her if she made contact?
- How would you feel if you heard that your client had been taken into hospital as a result of injecting heroin?

Summary

Dan begins by talking about his alcohol use, and his early use of aerosols. This leads him into memories that he does not disclose, but he experiences a panic attack. Jeannie helps him to relax. He doesn't talk about what caused it but talks about his relationship with Gemma, how he feels like a little boy with her. Then he talks of how boring his life is and feels overwhelmed by tiredness. He does not attend the next session. Jeannie gets a call from Dan's girlfriend, Gemma. He's injected and has been taken into hospital. She isn't too sure exactly what has happened.

CHAPTER 5

Making sense of the lapse

Session 7

Gemma had called again to say that Dan was back home, that he was OK and that
  he could make an appointment the following week for counselling.
Dan came in on time. Gemma had dropped him off and gone on to do some
  shopping.
'Hi Dan, come on through.'
'Thanks.'
'Seen Marie?'
'Yeah, she came out the day after I came home. Talked it through with her and,
  well, it's happened now. I'm glad to have come through it. Really shocked
  Gemma, and me.' Dan was shaking his head. 'Still feeling the effects. God my
  leg is sore.'
'What happened?' Jeannie didn't know the details, and wanted to give Dan the
  opportunity to tell her.

Jeannie could have maintained empathy and responded to the content of
what Dan had said. In some cases, the counsellor may know what has happened. She might have got some information from Marie, but here Jeannie
wants to get Dan's experience on events. If she simply told him she knew
what had happened it might block Dan from experiencing parts being heard
that he may not have told Marie. A person-centred counsellor who is aware
of events will let the client know this, but is likely to still ask what the client
may want to say about it in the context of the therapeutic relationship.

Dan told her how he had gone out for a drink with a mate he hadn't seen for a
  while on the Friday evening. 'Gemma was away for the weekend, visiting her
  sister. I didn't go. She felt she wanted some time with her and that was OK.
  It's not unusual or anything. So I went out with Rob, and, well, we had a few
  too many. Not good I know to be drinking while on the methadone, but I did.
  Seemed OK at the time. Got back home. Went to sleep OK. At least, I don't
  remember much. Got up next morning, well, quite late the next morning actually, and I guess I must have still been pretty much affected. Went to get my

methadone and dropped the bottle on the floor – stone floor, bottle smashed, glass, methadone everywhere. At first I panicked. Then I thought I'd be OK, I'd just drink more to get through the weekend. Thought that would work. It didn't.' Dan went quiet.

'So, it didn't hold you?'

Dan shook his head. 'No. At least, I don't think so. It's all very hazy now. I know I went out and got some strong lagers, thought that would do. I'm not sure after that. I think I must have drunk some and I guess, well, it didn't work. I felt bad by the evening, really bad. Tried to call a couple of people but couldn't get them. In the end went round to a guy I used to know, who deals. Kind of hoped he'd have methadone. Didn't want the heroin. But that was all he had, and there were a couple of others there who were jacking up, and I don't know, but I joined them. Couldn't get a vein up. Always did struggle. Went in the groin. Stayed there. Don't know how many times I jacked up. Think the alcohol had got to me as well. I was out of it, you know, really out of it.'

Jeannie sat giving Dan her full and undivided attention. It can't be easy for him to tell me all this, she thought. She was right.

'I feel awful. I thought I was over all of that. But once I started I just continued. I knew I had to get back though for Gemma, so I took some back with me, intended to smoke it, but I'd kept the needle I'd used and ended up injecting again on the Sunday as well. I was at least feeling a little better by the time Gemma got back, thought I could bluff my way through it. Thought she wouldn't notice. Thought I could get through to Monday and call here.'

Dan went silent again. Jeannie sensed the real struggle that was going on inside him. 'It's a real struggle to say these things, yeah?'

Dan nodded. 'I didn't get here Monday. I had enough left for the day so I used it. Thought I'd cleaned the needle. I was careful, real careful, I thought. Didn't go to work, though. Went out, just hung around, went back to where I'd got the gear, jacked up again and bought some more. Man, I was in another place. It had got hold of me again, really had. So fucking quick. So fucking quick. Anyway, knew my leg was a bit sore, swollen up a bit, but didn't think much of it, got home that afternoon, sat down and everything started spinning. Gemma didn't know what I'd been doing. I couldn't bring myself to tell her. She looked at my leg, it was getting more and more swollen and sore, and phoned the GP. I still couldn't tell her what I'd done. Just felt so ashamed, so guilty. I couldn't tell her, Jeannie, I couldn't tell her. Anyway, the doctor said he was on his way. By the time he arrived, I was in so much pain. I did tell him that I'd injected, what had happened. He wasn't too happy but called for an ambulance and they came and took me in. I don't remember much after that. But they told me later that I had a DVT – a deep-vein thrombosis – caused probably by the crap that had been cut into the gear, or by the needle that I was reusing. Anyway, they kept me in for a few days. Got me on a drip, got me stable again, and let me out at the end of the week.'

'Sounds awful.'

'Yeah, horrible. God, my leg, the pain. If that doesn't stop me, nothing will. I know now that I have to get clean, have to get away from the methadone and the alcohol. I don't want to risk that happening again, and I'm working on it with Marie. She wants me to be stable on the methadone for a couple more weeks or so and they have got me into their day programme to support me to keep me off the alcohol. I dried out while I was in, and she got it organised once she knew what was going on.'

You were lucky, Jeannie thought, not every area has a service like this. Some have so little service for people with alcohol problems, all the money seemingly going into drug services all the time. And not everyone can offer a day programme of support. So she was glad that Dan was using this.

'Off work then?'

'Yeah, doctor has signed me off for two weeks and, well, we'll see.'

'Mhmmm. So what now?'

'I need to earn Gemma's trust again. She's been good but she was really shocked. It helped her being there when Marie came round, helped her to understand how fast things can happen. I wouldn't have believed it but I guess I was up for it, and the alcohol probably left me thinking crazy ideas. I was out of it, just wasn't thinking properly. And it all went horribly wrong. And ...' Dan took a deep breath and put his head in his hands. He could feel the tears burning hot in his eyes, and the dampness spreading as they seeped through his fingers. 'Awful, Jeannie.' He took another deep breath. 'Fucking nightmare.' He continued to sit with his head in his hands.

Jeannie thought about reaching out to him, did a quick reality check and decided it was her need, that she wasn't sure what to do and felt she needed to do something. She could sense the pain Dan was experiencing although she knew it was her imagination. She couldn't feel what he was feeling. Slowly she spoke, seeking to convey her empathy not just in the words but through her tone of voice. 'Yeah. Says it all. Fucking nightmare.'

Dan began to sob. The tears felt heavier somehow and his throat began to burn. His chest was heaving as he breathed, each breath punctuated by tremors across his chest. It continued for some minutes. Jeannie didn't say anything; there seemed nothing more to say. Dan was experiencing his feelings, now, in the room, within their relationship. She felt her own breathing slow and deepen. She thought of saying something, but every phrase that went through her head felt all wrong – so many tears, so much hurt, I'm here for you. They all felt too trite and kind of patronising.

By being absorbed in her own thoughts about what to say, or not say, Jeannie has actually lost touch with the client. She is therefore being affected in some way by the silence such that she is finding it difficult to simply be with her client, something that can be extremely difficult and requires concentration and focus, and a disciplined approach to counselling.

Minutes passed. Jeannie had brought her focus back to Dan, seeking to be open to her own experiencing once more in relation to her contact with him. The idea of being trapped emerged for her, well, not so much an idea, as it didn't feel like a thought, more of a sense. She couldn't really define it but it felt very present to her. A phrase just came to mind, quite naturally and easily, and it had such a feeling of 'rightness' about it. She voiced it. 'Trapped in a nightmare.'

She waited. She had noticed Dan take a deeper, heavier breath just after she had spoken. She took this to indicate communication. She waited again, this time feeling more comfortable in herself. It seemed that by voicing that feeling, sense, whatever it was, she had somehow reaffirmed some kind of connection with Dan and what he was experiencing.

'Yeah. That's what it feels like. And I've been there a long, long time.' Dan spoke slowly and deliberately and with great intensity.

The atmosphere in the room felt electric to Jeannie. Again words formed without her needing to give them thought. She allowed them to be voiced. 'Too long.'

'Far too long.' The response was instant from Dan. 'Far too long.' As he spoke the second time the words were much slower and more deliberate. It seemed to Jeannie that he was talking to himself, telling himself that he had been trapped in the nightmare far too long. Yet she also recognised that this wasn't a case of words forming instinctively; she was putting them together and it wasn't the same. They were not coming out of her sensed connection with Dan in the same way that her earlier responses had. So she did not voice them, leaving Dan with whatever he was thinking and experiencing in response to his own voicing to himself of his recognition that he had been trapped in a nightmare for far too long.

The silence hung, but not heavily. It continued for some minutes.

Silences can be extremely productive. On the outside they seem to simply be that, a silence, but they can be working or processing silences. Dan is not just sitting, he is in process in the silence, and Jeannie respects this, indeed empathises with the presence of the process, and allows it to take Dan where he needs to be taken within the silence.

Jeannie held her focus and maintained her experienced attitude of warmth and unconditional positive regard for Dan. She believed that its presence had an effect, that we could, in some subtle way, pick up on how people are feeling towards us. She wanted to maintain this, offer this to Dan, letting him know that she cared about him in his struggle, within the process that was occurring inside him as he sat there now, his head still in his hands. He was not sobbing any more. There seemed to be a reoccurrence of a quality of stillness once more, like in that earlier session.

'There is something in me that knows I am more than all of this, and I need to hold on to that, I *need* to. I'm more than my drug use, I know I am, but how easy it is to slide back into it all again. Like stepping on an icy slope, one minute you are standing there, the next minute you've gone. But I have got to control this, I've got to.' As he spoke his voice got stronger and he took his hands away from his face, clenching his fists. 'This is a battle for my life, Jeannie, and I know that may sound overly dramatic, but that is how it feels. I am fighting for my life, for *my* life, for me, for who I am.' He lifted his head and looked into Jeannie's eyes. 'I have to come through this, I can't slip up again.'

Jeannie was struck by the power of Dan's voice and the forcefulness and determination in his eyes. It wasn't that they were staring, but they just seemed utterly determined, and in that moment she had no doubt that he would succeed. She had no reason to feel or experience this, but it was there, very present for her. She had learned to trust such profound inner prompting when it occurred, for it did feel connected to some deeper level of being.

'I am experiencing absolutely no doubt that you will.' Jeannie held his gaze. The moment lasted and lasted ... Two people connected in a common acknowledgement. Dan could feel himself absolutely still and centred, and utterly full of a will to succeed. He hadn't felt like this before; it was so powerful. Somehow, he knew. Yet it was a kind of knowing that didn't seem to attach itself to anything. He just knew, and that was enough.

Jeannie was also experiencing a similar response. Yet it felt like a quiet will, purposeful and deep, very deep. She pushed aside the temptation to analyse it and simply stayed with it. The moment continued and somehow time seemed to dissolve. Dan began to nod, ever so slightly. He got up and reached over and took Jeannie by the hand. 'Thank you. Thank you for that.' He tightened his lips, let go of her hand and returned to his seat.

Jeannie also nodded. 'I think that was powerful for both of us, Dan, it felt very deep, very affirming and very purposeful.'

'Yes, and I can still feel it. It's like my senses have become crystal clear, and that's unusual, and I'm sort of surprised given what I've been through, but it's like the chemicals have been rolled aside in some way and I am experiencing myself clearly. It's a good feeling, but it's more than a feeling, it seems more in my head, like a kind of sharpness, a focus, like something powerful in me has kind of, I don't know, kind of come together in some way.'

Jeannie nodded. A phrase came to mind, from a book she had read some time back, but which had made an impression on her, about the philosophy of spiritual evolution, and it seemed somehow strangely applicable to what she had just experienced, '*will, love and energy co-ordinated*' (Bailey, 1974, p.128). Will, love and energy co-ordinated. She put her thoughts aside and responded to Dan. 'So it's a kind of sharpness centred more up here, a sense of something coming together.' Jeannie put her hands either side of her head.

'Yes, but very much focused inside my head, not outside where you have your hands. Really felt centred in myself, in my head. It's still there but it is fading a little as we speak.' He shook his head. 'I feel different, clearer, like ... like emerging from a kind of fog. And yet I know the fog is close, you know, like it's lurking there, waiting to encircle me again.'

'What does the clarity allow you to see, Dan?' As she asked the question Jeannie knew it was partly her sense of feeling she wanted to help Dan use the clarity to perhaps gain his own sense of something, maybe his vision for himself, or direction, or whatever.

> Jeannie has not responded to the presence of the fog, which is what Dan was focusing on, and which was most present for him. Rather, she has felt moved to ask a question. She has stepped out of the client's frame of reference and yet if she is still profoundly connected with Dan then it is likely that her question will have meaning and relevance for him, and be somehow helpful. They have just come away from some kind of deep, maybe altered, state of consciousness. Rogers interestingly wrote of how in moments 'when I feel I am close to the transcendental core of me, I might behave in strange and impulsive ways in the relationship, ways which I cannot justify rationally, which have nothing to do with my thought processes. But these strange behaviours turn out to be right, in some odd way: it seems my inner spirit has reached out and touched the inner spirit of the other. Our relationship transcends itself and becomes part of something larger. Profound growth and healing energy are present' (Rogers, 1980, p.129).

She felt that while she couldn't justify her question, it somehow felt the right thing to say. It still felt disciplined and connected to Dan's experiencing and yet she knew how it could appear from outside that she was just saying whatever she happened to think of, ignoring the need for empathy. Yet she felt she knew herself well enough to be able to sense when an urge to say something was proceeding out of her sense of relatedness to, and presence with, Dan.

'I see a path, a straight path, and it leads towards a mountain. It's weird, I really can see it, Jeannie, like I am aware of you but just to your right, my left of you, I can see it, like a film projection on the wall. And I'm not tripping. And it leads towards this mountain and I know I am going to climb that mountain, I know it. It's like it's calling me, no, feels like a magnet pulling me. I have to head that way, I have to. And I can't look back. I can't look back.'

'You have to keep going forward, you can't look back.'

'No, but it's there, I can see it, so clear. Blue sky, green grass either side of the path, then the trees at the foot of the mountain and as it gets higher it becomes rocky. Yeah, wow, that's some, phew, I don't know what it is.' Dan realised that it had faded, he was just looking at the wall again. 'I've got to put the past behind me, Jeannie, and get on with my life. I have to. I'm going to. I'm going to stay dry on the alcohol and hold the methadone, and then look to reduce it. I want this clarity.'

'I really sense your excitement and energy, Dan, you really want to keep hold of this clarity.'

'Yeah.' He grinned and glanced at the clock.

Jeannie noticed. 'Yes, that time again.'

The session drew to a close and they agreed the time for the session the following week. Dan left feeling positive again, but it had been quite a roller coaster of a session. But something had shifted inside himself. He hoped it would last, he really did, but he knew that it was probably unlikely. But he could hope. And he had time off work now to get his head together and to really use the day programme. Yes, he was going to get through all this.

Jeannie sat and thought about the session that had just ended. She felt very sharp as well, as if that profound sense of connection had had a similar effect on both of them. Well, she thought to herself, I do wonder sometimes who gets most out of these sessions. A relationship is such a two-way process, and if there is deep connection one way then it seems reasonable that it is present the other way too. And if it is a growthful experience for the client it is very likely to have some kind of growthful effect on the therapist too. What was it she had heard someone once say, 'We get the clients we need.' She smiled at the thought. Seems to be a lot of truth in that.

Session 8

Dan had arrived early and was sitting in the waiting room when Jeannie came out a couple of minutes before the session was due to start. 'Oh, hi Dan, do you want to come through now?'

'Yes, thanks, I need to talk about something.' He walked ahead of her towards the room with a real air of purpose. It was very different to his usual manner, and certainly different to when he came in last session, when he was very subdued.

'So, what's on your mind?'

He grimaced. 'That image last week, you know, the path and the mountain, yeah?'

'Yeah, I remember you describing it.'

'Well, I dreamed about it, in fact I've dreamed about it a few times this week, but it's not just been about that mountain. You remember I said about not looking back?'

'Yeah, I think you said something like "I can't look back"?'

'Yeah, well in the dream I did. It was like I was pulled around.' Dan felt the goosebumps breaking out on his neck and back, and spreading down his arms and legs. He grimaced again, tightening his lips. 'Well ...' He stopped again, finding it difficult to say what he wanted, well, no, knew that he had to say. 'There's something I haven't told you, and, well, I nearly did but I stopped myself. It's like, well, it's just too damn painful. But I know now that I have to talk about it.'

Jeannie nodded, not wanting to interrupt Dan's flow.

Dan is finding his voice about something that is difficult for him to talk about, but he is talking and Jeannie wisely recognises the importance of minimal responses to allow him to continue. She certainly doesn't want to say something to disrupt him at this crucial time.

'It happened a long time ago. And I need to say this because of the image that kept coming back at me when I had the dream. I've never really talked about this to anyone before, and I know I'm going to find it hard, I can feel a lump in my throat already.'

Jeannie nodded again. 'Take your time.'

Dan went silent and Jeannie wondered if she had said the wrong thing. Maybe she had disturbed his flow after trying to be careful not to.

'When I was nine or maybe ten, can't remember for sure, back in the days when we were sniffing glue and gas, well, we were messing about one day and ...' Dan stopped. The image of Billy's face had invaded his thoughts again. He took a deep breath, but he could feel his throat tighten as he tried to continue. 'Billy was a friend of mine, known him, well, ever since I went to school.' He stopped again, he could feel tears coming into his eyes. He blinked. 'Sorry, this is hard, shit this is hard.'

Jeannie tightened her lips and nodded. 'Yeah.'

Dan took another deep breath. 'Well, there was this one time ...' Dan could feel his throat tighten again and the tears starting to escape from his eyes; he couldn't stop them. He knew this was going to happen. He'd lived with it so many years, keeping it at bay, using ... using anything to keep himself away from the memory, from the feelings, from the pain. He couldn't say anything, the tears just continued down his face. 'I can't get his face out of my head, Jeannie, all these years and it's still there.'

'Billy.'

'Yeah, Billy.' Dan closed his eyes and shook his head again, tightening his lips and his jaw as he did so. He lifted his left hand up to his mouth.

Jeannie sat and stayed with Dan, aware of his movements, his expression, like she was finely tuned, yet aware that she hadn't a clue what he had to tell her. But that didn't matter. He was where he was, struggling to voice something that had been with him for about 20 years, something he didn't talk about, something painful, something that had left him with an image of Billy's face seared into his soul.

Dan closed his eyes again and the tears trickled down his face, dropping from his cheeks on to the collar of his shirt, creating two darkening spots that slowly spread. His breath started to tremor and Jeannie's thoughts momentarily went back to that panic attack in the earlier session. Had that been some kind of a bodily reaction linked to this memory? She pushed the thought aside. She'd lost Dan again; she needed to give him her attention.

Dan had opened his eyes and was looking at Jeannie. 'He died, Jeannie, he died, right there in front of us. He died.' He closed his eyes again, more tears fell, and he screwed up his eyes. 'Why did he have to die, why him? I loved him, Jeannie, we were so close, like twin brothers, and I can see his face. His lips swollen and blue, his whole face blue, staring, staring. And I didn't know what to do, none of us did. We had all been laughing and fooling around with the gas and some aerosol. I don't know exactly what he did, we thought he was fooling around. We laughed at him, Jeannie, we laughed at him, and he was dying.' The tears poured out of Dan and he collapsed into a heap in the chair, his left arm across his stomach supporting his right elbow, his right hand across his face.

'I laughed at him, the last thing he must have seen was me, laughing at him.' He covered his face with both his hands. 'Oh God, oh God, what have I done? What have I done?'

Jeannie picked up on the shift to the present, or at least that Dan was talking as if it was happening now. She felt the waves of emotion, the deep sadness, the hurt, the horror of it all. She realised that she had closed her own eyes and also felt tears escaping. She opened them and looked straight into Dan's very red and watery eyes staring back at her. 'The horror of that realisation.'

Dan nodded and again lifted his right hand up to his chin. 'I didn't know what to do. I didn't know what to do. When we realised, we panicked. We just panicked. We ran off, we ran off and left him.'

Jeannie responded in a way that acknowledged what was being said but sought to hold Dan on his experience.'Ran away, didn't know what to do, so many feelings, but didn't know what to do.'

'No, it was horrible, seeing him lying there. It was so quick, we tried to rouse him, but he wasn't breathing, he couldn't breathe. We didn't understand. And his eyes, staring ...' Tears flowed once more as Dan put his head back in his hands, his body convulsing with the pain of his emotion. 'I can't get that image out of my head.'

'Just keep seeing Billy's face, his eyes ...'

Dan stayed silent. He had never felt like this before, even when his brother had died he had never felt like this. He felt ... he didn't know what he felt, but he knew it hurt and it seemed to fill the whole of his upper body. His arms and legs were heavy; he just felt like one huge bubble of hurt; he felt himself screwing up his eyes once again as another wave of emotion hit him. He couldn't think about what was happening to him, he was just overwhelmed. He couldn't believe how much emotion he had. He took a deep breath and rubbed his eyes. 'Have I been carrying this all my life?'

Jeannie nodded. 'Probably, and maybe there are other tears you haven't cried in there as well, about other painful experiences.'

'Yeah. I have never really showed my feelings. I've always controlled them with the drugs, but I can't do that any more. I have to face them, don't I? I guess that means more of this, perhaps, or does it all go in one go?' He shook his head. 'No, I know it is going to take longer, and that's fucking terrifying, and yet, I know I must face it, face myself.'

Jeannie really sensed the terror that was present for Dan and she acknowledged this, using his words. She agreed that it was himself he was having to face. Dan nodded, blew his nose and dried his eyes. He sat, breathing deeply for a while, regaining his composure.

'Well, I've made a start. I've shared something with you that no one else has heard me describe, not since it happened anyway. And no one has witnessed my pain.' His eyes began to water again.

> Sometimes it can seem that the counsellor is offering a process of bearing witness to the client, and more particularly to the experience that the client is describing or reacting to. This very process can be intensely therapeutic. The client feels that his experience is somehow validated, that however horrible it is, another person has been prepared to stay with him. He is therefore not so alone with it; it has been shared, heard and the person who has listened continues to accept him warmly.

'First time anyone has witnessed your pain – I feel privileged, Dan, I really do.' Jeannie really meant this. On a number of occasions she had heard clients tell her things that had been locked up for years. Things that so often involved pain and shame. She always regarded these experiences of listening as precious, to be treated with tremendous respect.

'Thanks.' Dan sat for a few moments. He was thinking now about what happened afterwards, and realised he needed to continue with what happened. He had started but it was only half the story, and while what followed hadn't felt so dramatic, it hadn't been very pleasant. 'I need to say more. I need to talk about what followed. I feel like I am halfway through a journey with you here and I need to complete it. You don't need to say anything, I think I just need you to listen.'

'OK.'

> Jeannie respects Dan's need to just talk. She is empathising with his wishes and she allows him to speak at his own pace, without interruption.

'We all left Billy, and headed off to Peter's house, which was closest. We were all, I guess, in shock. His father was there and heard us come in and saw immediately from the looks on our faces and the state we were in that something had happened. He asked us what it was. We all looked at each other, and I remember thinking that it was Peter's dad and he should say something. I nudged him. "It's Billy, dad, we didn't do anything, we were just messing about, we didn't do anything." With that he burst into tears. Peter's dad asked us where Billy was and we told him. He asked what happened; we told him. He looked terribly shaken; the colour drained from his face. He grabbed the phone and called 999. After telling them what had happened he came with us to where Billy was. None of us wanted to get close. Peter's dad went over to him.' Dan stopped speaking; Jeannie sat quietly waiting for him to continue.

Dan continued, describing how the ambulance and the police had arrived, how they had had to go down to the police station and tell them what had happened. The events that followed, the funeral, the inquest. 'I should have done something, but I couldn't, Jeannie, I couldn't. It was my fault, it was all my fault.'

'You really blame yourself for it, Dan, but once Billy had used the gas or the aerosol, there would have been nothing you could have done.'

'I know, I know. I can accept that now. I understand what happens, how it freezes the respiratory system. I know now that I couldn't have saved him, but at the time . . . at the time . . .' Dan put his head in his hands again, drew them down to his mouth and blew out a deep breath.

'It feels really weird talking about all this, after so many years. Yet it feels so real; it doesn't seem so long ago and yet I know that it was. My feelings and memories are so real, so close. I couldn't have done anything, I realise that now. Not after it happened. Just one sniff too many; I guess I should have learned from that but I never did. Stopped me using solvents though, never sniffed again after that. But I did drink, we all did. And then, well, you know the rest. Felt so bad, over the years, and trying to push the memory away.' As he spoke those last words his voice weakened and his eyes watered again. 'So guilty, I've felt so guilty for so long. I'd push it away, bury it, but it came back, it always came back.'

'The guilt wouldn't go away.' Jeannie appreciated that Dan having blamed himself, thinking he could have done something to help Billy, left him feeling guilty.

Dan shook his head. 'It's been there with me for so long. Knowing what really happened, why he died, doesn't make any difference though. Doesn't make any difference at all.' Jeannie knew she was now feeling puzzled. And yet she also recognised how such a powerfully traumatic experience could leave somebody unable to change their feelings or beliefs associated with the event.

'He still died. The knowledge you have doesn't alter that.'

Dan breathed deeply again and sighed in response. 'I will regret to the end of my life what happened, and I will never forgive myself. Never forgive myself.'

Jeannie felt somehow something wasn't right, but she couldn't make sense of it. Dan was blaming himself, feeling guilt, seemingly to her indicating that he felt responsible for Billy's death. She appreciated how as a child he would very likely have felt that way, but now? Something didn't feel right, but she couldn't grasp what it was, and she was aware that her train of thought had taken her away from listening to Dan, and the burden of guilt he was carrying.

Jeannie is troubled; something isn't feeling quite right somehow but she does not know what it is. Does she voice this, or bring her attention back to Dan, noting her feelings and waiting to see what emerges? She is unsure of herself and chooses not to say anything, deciding instead to place her prime emphasis on her empathy for Dan, on listening to what else he needs to say.

'Never, ever forgive yourself, that feels a huge burden to carry for the rest of your life.'

'Yeah, but I have got a life, Billy hasn't.'

'Mhmmm.'

'Why did I do it?' Dan paused, his eyes looking straight into Jeannie's, as if he wanted her to have an answer for him. 'Why?'

Jeannie assumed he was talking about the sniffing. She felt a pull to answer but resisted it, and responded with an empathic reflection. 'You really want an answer to that "Why?"'

Dan nodded. 'Just did it, we had all brought something that day, except Billy. I'd managed to nick this lighter fuel, the others had just brought glue.' Dan paused.

Jeannie now knew what hadn't been making sense and now made absolute sense. Oh God, she thought, oh no, carrying that around with him all these years, oh no. She spoke slowly, partly because she could sense the immensity of what she was saying, and partly because she knew she was checking it out, although she now knew the reality before she spoke.

'It was your lighter fuel.'

Dan nodded slightly and slowly. 'Yeah. If it hadn't been for me, maybe he'd still be alive.'

'And you blame yourself and have been carrying the guilt, locked up inside you, ever since?'

'Yeah. And I can't bear it any more. I'm tired of it and yet I cannot forgive myself. His eyes, they were a bright, watery blue, big, round. He had wonderful eye-lashes, had never noticed them before, and I can see them so clearly, his body twitching, his mouth open but nothing happening. No air going in or coming out. Nothing. And going slowly more and more blue. And I, we, laughed at him.' Dan took a deep breath, lifted his left hand to his mouth and looked to the ceiling. 'So you see, I killed him. I killed my best friend, Jeannie, I killed my best friend.'

Jeannie looked at him and felt a huge wave of sadness for this little boy who had internalised such a terrifying belief about what he had done, and therefore about himself. A sentence was immediately in her mind, but she did not voice it: and you've been punishing yourself ever since. In and out of prison, taking risks with his body with the drugs. She wondered what had happened after the event? She guessed he hadn't felt punished, or punished enough, that he had to maybe punish himself. She brought her thinking back; this was all speculation, she needed to stay with Dan. She had lost contact with him at a crucial moment, voicing his belief that he had killed his best friend.

Within the counselling relationship there are often really key moments when powerful disclosures are made, and the response that the counsellor makes is crucial. Rather like in tennis, if that isn't stretching metaphors a bit far, the really good players tend to win the big points, points that win, or save, games and sets. The most effective person-centred counsellor will recognise the big disclosures (which may be a single word spoken very quietly), the moments of deep connection, and will convey to the client in an appropriate and meaningful way their empathic understanding of what is being communicated, their warm acceptance towards the client, and will be genuine and authentic in that moment.

'I feel so much sadness as you tell me this; you have carried this for so long, that you killed Billy.'

Dan felt heard. He felt that his deep secret was being respected; it somehow made it feel a little easier. Yeah, he thought, yeah, she accepts what happened and how I feel about it. He took a deep breath again.

Another counsellor might have contradicted Dan, trying to rescue him from his anguish by saying that he was only a child, he didn't know any better, that it was an accident, anything to make Dan (and probably more likely the counsellor) feel better, rather than sit with the uncomfortable reality in Dan's mind that he, and he alone, had killed his best friend.

Staying with the client's frame of reference is crucial and a feature of person-centred working, coupled with a deep trust that whatever the client's beliefs, they will be therapeutically assisted by being heard and taken seriously. Dan is talking about experiences and feelings that he has disclosed to no one else. To try to change what he has felt for so long would undermine him and would be likely to be extremely damaging, maybe leaving him unwilling to say anything again for a long time, and certainly not with any counsellor who tried to take him away from his own experience. The person-centred counsellor is not seeking to change the client, but to attend to him or her, to listen to what they have to say, to offer the necessary and sufficient conditions and allow the client's own inner process to help them move towards a more constructive way of being, reflecting an increasingly congruent sense of self.

Jeannie allowed the silence that had begun to continue. Dan had looked down, and had begun to tap and rub his fingertips together. Whatever must he be feeling, she thought to herself. She knew she couldn't begin to gain a sense of this from her own experience; she needed Dan to show her.

'I know you can't take this away from me, and I don't want you to. This experience is part of who I am, but I am glad you know it now.'

'So am I Dan, so am I.' She said the words slowly and looked into his eyes as she spoke. She knew she really meant it. So did Dan.

This is a key response: not a moment for some sickly-sweet response in typically immature counselling language such as, 'and I am so very glad that you have told me this', delivered from the textbook and not from the heart.

These are very human moments that Jeannie and Dan are sharing, moments of therapeutic intimacy. The need for authenticity is absolutely vital. The mature person-centred counsellor will have cultivated the necessary self-awareness and discipline to be able to offer this.

The session slowly drew to a close. Jeannie checked that Dan was feeling OK enough in himself to head off, and he said that he was, that he felt a lot lighter in himself and that he had taken a big step in that session. He thanked Jeannie again, holding her hand as he did so and looking into her eyes. They ended up giving each other a hug, and he thanked her again as he left the room. Jeannie followed him to the exit; she felt unable to just turn and leave him to make his own way out. She watched him leave before turning and slowly walking back to her room. She felt she had a lot to think about, and a lot to process. She was glad that her next supervision session wasn't far away. She knew she was very concerned that she had felt she had lost contact with Dan when he had disclosed his belief that he had killed Billy. She would have to carry her thoughts and her feelings for a couple more days.

After writing her notes and spending a little more time thinking about Dan, and what he had carried for so long, and intended to continue carrying, she realised that she needed to get ready to go. She didn't have another client that evening, which she was grateful for. She would have had to have gone out for a breath of fresh air or something if she had, to give herself a sense of having a clear transition between clients. She left, headed back to her car, and as she sat down behind the steering wheel she found herself suddenly taken by a wave of emotion. What she had just been hearing, the stark reality of it all, suddenly just hit her: a nine-year-old little boy living in a house where his father got drunk regularly, where he and his brothers would huddle together during the fights downstairs, had internalised the belief that he had killed his best friend.

Points for discussion

- Consider the difference between 'being with' someone in silence and 'waiting for' someone in silence to speak.
- What for you were the key moments in Sessions 7 and 8, and why?
- Why do you feel Dan has chosen this time to disclose his childhood experience of Billy's death?
- What were your personal reactions to reading through Sessions 7 and 8? How were you affected and how might this impact on your work if you had been Dan's counsellor?
- Do you feel Jeannie was appropriate in her responses to Dan within these sessions according to person-centred theory of offering the core conditions of empathy, unconditional positive regard and congruence?
- Reading the final paragraph, how were you left feeling?
- How would you deal with the feelings that arose in Jeannie after Session 8 had finished?

Summary

Dan describes what happened leading up to his injecting and being taken to hospital, and the part alcohol played in it. He feels it all as a nightmare that he has been in far too long. Jeannie allows him to stay in a silence; he becomes emotional and it leads to him affirming his need to come through it, that there is more to him than his drug use. He finds clarity emerging within him and has a metaphorical vision. The following session he describes the death of his friend, Billy, in childhood, and how it left him feeling so guilty. He discloses how he has never spoken to anyone before about it in the way that he has with Jeannie, who, after the session, is herself affected by a wave of emotion.

CHAPTER 6

Supervision 2

'I need some time today on Dan, my new client at the agency that I spoke about a
   month ago.'
'Yes, I remember, on methadone and trying to move on, but with a long history of
   using all kinds of substances, but generally suppressants.'
'Yes. Well, a lot has happened, Max, and it is hard to know where to begin.' She
   stopped and thought about it. She continued. 'In a way I really want to talk
   about me because I experienced a really powerful reaction to him after the last
   session, though I feel I need to explain what has been happening to put my
   reaction in context.'
Max nodded. 'So, major concern about a reaction that you had but it sounds like a
   lot has been going on.'
'That's an understatement!'
'Tell me about it.'
'Well, a few sessions back, probably the first after I saw you, he had a panic
   attack, and that was somewhat unnerving, and I remember a sense that somehow his body was trying to tell me something. Seemed like he was maybe getting close to something inside himself but was choosing not to talk about it, but
   his body was communicating huge amounts of anxiety. I highlighted it, offering him the opportunity to pick up on it, but he didn't. He wanted to emphasise
   his need to move on. I was left wondering if I should have held him on his bodily
   reaction a bit more, try to help him explore it, but I also know that I respect his
   choice to focus on what is important to him, and maybe at that time he just
   wasn't in a place to do that. I now believe that this was the case, and it was
   right to let it go and stay with him.'

The person-centred counsellor would expect to stay with the client, only
voicing their own feelings, reactions, thoughts or perceptions where they
were strong and persistent, and were genuinely felt to be emerging as a
result of their contact and communication with the client. It is possible for
a client to consistently speak in ways that are incongruent to their body language, for instance someone describing themselves as feeling relaxed or OK
about something when in fact their body is strained and they are constantly
moving their hands in an anxious and distracting manner.

In such instances, the client is communicating two experiences, and the person-centred counsellor can helpfully empathise with both, not necessarily pointing out the contradiction, which would be an interpretation, but simply letting the client know what they are experiencing as being communicated to them. The client is thereby offered the opportunity to clarify their body language if they wish to. Either way, that part of them which is driving the body has an opportunity to feel heard and may then find its voice if the client's process allows it.

'Was this something you wondered at the time, or in hindsight? I am curious as to whether your experience was, if you like, in real time, in the moment of connecting with the client, or if it was in retrospect?'

'I thought about it at the time, but it didn't feel a big issue. I guess it was later that I began to wonder. He moved on to talk about something else, his girlfriend I think, I'm not sure now, and I guess it was after the session that I was aware that actually something that had seemed quite major had occurred but then been kind of left behind somehow. But things happened which provoked, maybe that's not the right word, but certainly encouraged Dan to disclose what I think may well have been behind the panic attack, although it is speculation.'

Max was intrigued. He was aware Jeannie was talking a lot but he wasn't really getting many facts. He wondered if it was a parallel process. He voiced his wondering.

Parallel processing is where a feature of the client's experiencing is played out within someone else. In this instance it is the content of what Jeannie is saying: Max is wondering if it is a parallel process, reflecting something of the way that the client presents his story. It can be useful to identify and work with as it can often shed light on what may be present for the client. It is often indicative of a powerful dynamic being present within the client. Working with it in supervision can highlight how much the counsellor has been drawn into this dynamic which could impact on their ability to be congruent or block accurate empathy.

'I sort of have this feeling that you are saying a lot but not telling me much. Lots of references to things happening but not sure what they are yet, and I know you are getting to them, but I am wondering if this process is actually reflecting something about the client, or your relationship with the client.'

Jeannie thought about it. Lots of words but not much information. She reflected back on what she knew about Dan. She knew of some key events in his life, and she had experienced being with him while he experienced the deep hurt, the sense of guilt, of anxiety that had emerged in the sessions. Max was right. She knew a little, but there were big gaps. She knew nothing about his prison experiences, of his early childhood, well, not much about his teenage years either other than references to his drug use and obviously the impact of the death of his brother. But yes, Max was right, she didn't know much although she felt she had experienced such a lot with Dan. Curious, she thought.

What Jeannie has recognised is important. She has a concept of having con-nected with Dan, she has a lot to talk about and yet there is so much of him that she is unaware of. Maintaining her false sense of their relationship might block exploring the areas that are currently invisible to her. She needs to be open to an awareness that there is more, much more, to Dan than what she has experienced so far.

'There are big gaps, a lot I don't know about him, and yet at another level, at a feeling level, I really do feel I have connected deeply with him and do know him. But there is a kind of split here somehow. Or is it just that we have only had eight, no, seven sessions, he didn't attend one, and there was the session he was stoned. But no, it's like I have kind of snapshots of events, pretty traumatic events, but specific events in his life.' She paused and thought about it some more. 'Maybe that's how it is for Dan. Maybe he isn't connected with every-thing that has happened, bits forgotten, and he is giving me himself in the way that he experiences himself. I hadn't thought of that. But it makes sense the more I think about it.'

Max wanted to encourage Jeannie to think about the implications this had for their relationship and the work they were doing. He asked about this.

Jeannie felt that maybe Dan would begin to make connections, in a sense begin to perhaps join up the events and how they impacted on him. 'He's wary, isn't he?' she suddenly said. 'He is taking time to trust me, telling me what he feels able to allow me to hear, at least that's maybe how it started. I think that is changing. I think, I know, he is now telling me things that he knows he has to say, that he needs to say. He's not controlling his disclosures the same – and control must be big for him – because, well, let me explain what happened. He dropped his methadone over a weekend after drinking too much the night before, and ended up injecting heroin, for what seemed like at least a couple of days, tried to avoid telling his girlfriend, but ended up developing a deep-vein thrombosis in his leg – he'd injected in the groin. Put him in hospital. And he also had a really deep experience as well, a kind of vision of a mountain he was being drawn towards, happened in the session, then he dreamt about it but it was different and it made him realise he had something he needed to talk about. We had a couple of really deep connections, felt spiritual. But anyway, what came out of the last session was that when he was about nine his best friend died in front of him, respiratory failure as a result of sniffing some kind of sol-vent, and he blames himself for his death – he had got the stuff that Billy, his friend, had sniffed. Watched him go blue and die in front of him. Has carried it around in his head for years, telling no one what he felt, and clearly has used substances to try and blot it out. And I think he has been punishing himself as well, maybe that's part of his drug use, and getting into prison, I don't know, I may be running ahead on that. He hasn't made that connection and I'm not going to suggest it.'

Counselling, and particularly person-centred counselling, is not about making connections for the client. It is better for them to be supported through their own process of making sense of themselves. The offering of the core conditions facilitates this process, by offering an atmosphere in which the client gradually feels freer to move around within themselves, where their conditions of worth are less actively dominant and they can begin to take often tentative steps towards developing a fresh perspective on themselves and their past and present experiences.

'No, that would certainly be outside of a person-centred way of working. He has to be allowed to move at his own pace, make his own connections when he is able to.'

Jeannie nodded. 'Yeah, I know.' She yawned. 'Gee, I feel tired all of a sudden.' She yawned again. 'Oh, sorry, it's just come over me.' She yawned again, and again, and again. 'My eyes suddenly feel really gritty.'

'Really gritty.'

Jeannie nodded.

'Something's leaving or making you really tired, yes, so what were we saying, or were you thinking or experiencing just before it started?'

Perhaps Max should have simply stayed with Jeannie in her tiredness rather than directing her back to what they had been discussing. This would have arguably been a more person-centred response.

'I made the comment about him maybe punishing himself.' As she said it she felt another yawn coming on, a really big one, forcing her to really open her mouth wide. 'Oh dear.' She promptly yawned again, feeling the back of her jaw straining as she did so. 'God, I'm so tired.'

'Tired of?'

'I don't know. I know I'm the one that's tired, but am I tired of Dan? I don't think so. I feel really touched by what he has gone through, and I really am wanting to be there for him and help him make sense of it all and move on. I feel, I was feeling, quite energised, although quite sad as well when I think about his early life. But I . . . I don't feel tired of him, and yet . . . oh here I go again.' Another big yawn, and another. 'Are you feeling tired?'

Max wasn't. 'No, and your yawns don't seem to be provoking yawns in me, which is unusual because they often seem strangely contagious.'

'So it has to be me, but I'm not aware of anything I'm tired of. Could I be tuning into Dan? What was it we were saying, about . . .' She thought back. 'Yes, I was speculating about whether he was . . . ,' another yawn, 'punishing himself,' another yawn. 'That's it. He is tired of punishing himself, or maybe part of him,' another yawn, 'is tired of,' another yawn, 'punishing himself. Maybe that's why he told me about Billy's death, maybe he's tired of carrying around the memory and the guilt, even though he also told me that he would never forget it and would blame himself for the rest of his life, at least, I think that's what he said. Something like that, anyway.'

Jeannie closed her eyes; it felt good. 'He's at risk, Max; he may not simply be tired of carrying his feelings and memories, maybe he wants to close his eyes to it all, and the way he has always done that is with drugs. Oh shit, I know this may seem crazy, but I think he's at risk of another lapse, even though he wants to get free of the drugs and the alcohol – yes, he said he stopped sniffing after Billy died, but began using alcohol to help him forget it, blot it out, dull his feelings. So alcohol he associates with dealing with Billy while heroin is associated with dealing with his brother, at least injecting heroin, he was already smoking it. No, it started him smoking. I think that's how it was. Again, bits.'

Max was stuck with something and unclear. He felt he needed clarity. 'I feel a bit lost on why you are saying you feel he is at risk.'

'The sense that if he is tired of it all but cannot get rid of it by talking it through and out, by releasing feelings, he may go back to substances. But that's obvious. I think I'm losing the plot here, getting myself tangled up.'

'It is complex, Jeannie, lots of threads and at the moment it seems that Dan hasn't got them connected.'

'I guess I'm struggling with it too.'

Max was suddenly aware that Jeannie hadn't yawned for while. 'You're not yawning.'

'No, I'm not, am I? So what happened here? Recognising the complexity, the risk? Talking has somehow released the tiredness? Is that what it's telling me, that talking it through may, for Dan, release his being tired of it all?'

'Speculation, but maybe. Something has happened. How are you feeling?'

'Different. Lighter. Less burdened somehow.' She shook her head. 'What was that all about?'

'I don't know, but it seems to have shifted something for you. Anything else changed?'

Jeannie did a reality check on herself. She brought Dan back to mind, and watched her reactions as she did so. She felt less anxious. She felt a kind of OKness about him, as if she knew all would be OK. Was she fooling herself, avoiding something, or was this genuine? It felt genuine. She described it to Max. 'I feel less burdened and have a sense that all will be OK with Dan. I can't give you a reason, but that's how I feel.'

'Less burdened by Dan?'

Jeannie smiled. 'Yes, that's got to be part of it, hasn't it? I had such a strong reaction after the last session; when I got back to my car to drive home, a wave of sadness hit me. Maybe I've been carrying Dan around with me more than I realised. Maybe he has affected me without me fully realising it. Not that I don't want to be affected, I do. I have to be affected to be effective, but maybe I need to talk things through more often; maybe I need supervision more regularly on this client.'

'Try to stop it building up?'

'Maybe. I'm concerned that if I am overloading without realising it then it may start to affect my ability to be with and stay with him. Stay with him. Shit. I lost him at a really critical moment, when he said about believing he killed Billy, I lost him. I felt my own sadness for him and ... oh yes, here we go, ended up speculating in my own mind about how he may be punishing himself. And that's what set me off here being tired, wasn't it? OK, so, something is happening in me making it difficult to hear Dan and it seems to be linked to profound sadness and the notion of self-punishment, and being tired of it all.'

Working with people who have been deeply affected by traumatic experiences, or who carry strong, emotional content, even when it is bottled up and not expressed, can threaten to overwhelm the person-centred counsellor who is seeking to maintain openness to their client and to their own experiencing. The need not only for regular, supportive supervision but also other recreational experiences is vitally important to enable the counsellor to unwind and dissipate emotional knots that can develop and block empathic sensitivity.

'So you lost your empathic rapport, unable to stay with him because of sadness and feeling tired?'

'No, I wasn't feeling tired at that time, just sadness and then thoughts about punishment. Let me think about this for a moment, and try and get a sense of what is present for me now.' Jeannie tried to reconnect with that sadness; she brought back to her mind that image of Dan as a boy, of the terror and the guilt, of having no one to talk to, of him and his brother huddled together at home ... She began to feel her eyes watering, and tears trickling down her cheeks. She felt a lump in her throat. She allowed the feelings to flow through her and the tears continued to trickle from her eyes. She screwed her eyes up as another wave of sadness and emotion hit her. It passed, and she felt relief. She swallowed and took a deep breath. 'I still don't know what this is about, other than maybe I simply feel affected by his story; it just feels so enormous, so overwhelming. I just can't really get a sense of exactly what it must be, or have been, like. Yeah, I cry tears for him, and I am glad to have released them. It isn't bringing anything personal up for me; I think I'm just very touched by his life, his struggle and the feelings he has kept to himself for so many years.'

'Yeah, he really has released sadness in you.'

'Yeah, and it's good to let it go. I needed to. I need to watch I don't build up again.' Jeannie took another deep breath. 'OK, I think that's what I needed.' She glanced up at the clock. 'That time already. OK, I think I'm clear for now, and, look, can I call you if I sense it's building up, or if I lose contact with Dan again in the session? I think I really need to have the possibility of extra support here if I need it, though maybe I have done enough for now.'

Max agreed to this, and they decided that Jeannie could call him if she needed to talk anything through, and if he couldn't talk at the time then they'd arrange a time for a phone call. That felt good, Jeannie thought, as she prepared to leave and head back home. She was so glad she worked in a profession in which supervision of this nature was part of the professional requirement to practise. Time to explore personal reactions was so precious, so important, both for her own well-being and to ensure that she was more likely to keep in contact with her clients during sessions. She didn't want to lose Dan again at a critical moment; he deserved better than that.

CHAPTER 7

'Parts' of Dan begin to emerge as he connects with his past

Session 9

Jeannie knew she felt a little different this week as she waited for Dan to arrive. She was now much more mindful of the impact he was having on her, and while she knew she needed to guard against her own struggle to contain it, she also recognised that she had to be open. In fact, since her supervision session, she had been reflecting more on this and in a way had reached the conclusion that perhaps she simply needed to make more visible the impact it was having on her to help make real the nature and extent of what Dan was bringing into the their relationship. It brought to mind the notion of transparency that she had read about many times as a way of describing an aspect of congruence, and the importance of self-acceptance. If she could not be accepting of her feelings and reactions to Dan, embrace them as part of the reality of her own process within their relationship, she was not going to be much help to him.

Jeannie was also mindful that, for her, being a person-centred counsellor was a process of personal development. She wanted to get to know herself and to move towards becoming that 'fully functioning person' that Rogers referred to. She needed to experience herself, and not only those elements of herself which clients brought to her attention through the therapeutic contact and process. There was also her own stuff, and she needed to be able to connect with that and be accepting of the difficult and uncomfortable parts of herself as much as those that made her feel good. She needed to be whole, open to her own experiencing, whatever it might be, and bring that whole person called Jeannie into relationship with her clients.

Mearns and Thorne highlight the importance of self-acceptance within the person-centred counsellor, stating that 'not to be self-accepting is to entertain a contradiction at the very centre of the therapeutic enterprise'. They go on to comment that such 'self-acceptance should not be confused with complacency or a kind of weary resignation' and that where this is the case,

> the 'person has usually called a halt to self-exploration' and is 'no longer growing and unlikely to assist the development of others' (1999, p.26).

So Jeannie sat in the counselling room feeling much more open to her feelings, and wanting to be as fully present as possible for Dan when he arrived.

He was a few minutes late, roadworks. He apologised and sat himself down.

'So, how do you want to use the time we have this evening?'

'I'm not sure, but I have a sense of wanting to explore more of the past and how it has affected me. I've been thinking during the week, and a lot of ideas have come out through the day programme, about how I carry chaos in my head and find it really hard to tolerate order, or just what other people might call normality, but that I am learning to do it, albeit slowly.'

'Mhmmm, so the day programme is giving you a clearer sense of your issues around chaos and order, yeah?'

'And how much effect it has had on me. I do find it hard to feel settled, and maybe part of that is the drugs, and being off the alcohol – which I'm managing OK so far, though it isn't easy – but I do seem to feel split, you know? Like there's a part of me wanting to just be normal, just get on with a routine life, working in the day, coming home, being with Gemma and her son, and just doing normal things together. Yet another part of me seems to really, I don't know how to describe it . . . finds it difficult, I suppose.'

'So, yes, feeling split, part of you really wanting the kind of normality you describe, and yet this other part that is somehow hard to describe, finding it all very difficult?' Jeannie voiced her empathic response as a question to maybe encourage a climate of exploration as she sensed Dan was wanting to make greater sense of this split in himself.

'There's something in me that makes it feel as though normal isn't normal. I don't think I'm making much sense.'

Jeannie found it very clear, and it was not uncommon, though she knew better than to make assumptions as to precisely what Dan meant based on other people's experiences. 'Sounds clear to me, that the normal you sense others as having, and that part of you wants, just doesn't feel normal. Does that convey what you are experiencing?' She made it sound more like a statement, then added the question to allow Dan to then decide whether what she had said rang true, or not.

'My normal's all wrong, and that just feels so scary, so fucking scary.'

> Here is a powerful recognition from Dan, and the response from Jeannie will be important. She actually responds to Dan's feelings rather than his insight. She could have responded to both, allowing Dan the choice as to which direction he wished to take, and arguably this could have been more person-centred. Clients experience thoughts and feelings within their inner frame of reference and the person-centred counsellor is there to listen to and accept both.

Jeannie had kind of picked up the notion that Dan's language tended to get more colourful as his feelings intensified, so she guessed that it was really scaring him. She empathised with it. 'It really does scare you, doesn't it, really is fucking scary.'

'Yeah. I mean, who am I, what am I, where am I going, where have I been? It's like everything suddenly feels very unsafe and, well, I was going to say fluid. Like I don't know what's solid, and the crazy thing is the only bit that feels really solid is the drugs, like, I know where I am with them, even though most of the time I was out of it. It's crazy. I'm confused.'

'It's crazy, you're confused.' Jeannie kept her empathy to his summary perception and the effect that this was having on Dan.

Dan sat quietly. 'I mean, just sitting here now, talking like this, I feel really anxious inside, like I need something to settle myself back down and I don't know how to do it, except with a drink or drugs. And I know I have other options, we've discussed them on the programme, but when it comes to it the only thought that comes to mind is taking something.'

'Taking something to take away the anxiety.'

'Yeah. And that's what I've always done, and what I still want to do, and it's not what I want to do as well. I feel like I've got the devil on one shoulder and, I don't know, some kind of angel on the other, and I'm in the middle and I'm confused.'

'Yeah, confused by the conflicting voices?'

'I don't know what to believe sometimes, and often I believe both and then I'm still stuck in the middle.'

Jeannie nodded. 'Not just stuck but stuck in the middle.'

Dan took a deep breath, yes, he thought, not just stuck, but stuck in the middle, that really does sum up where I am. Stuck in the middle, part of me telling me one thing, part of me saying another. And I end up believing them both. He sat in silence, pondering on it, feeling confused by it, getting more and more stuck with it.

Jeannie did not interrupt. She noted that every now and then Dan took a deep breath and sighed, like he was really struggling with something. She voiced it, speaking softly so as not to overly disturb Dan's process. 'Such a struggle within you.'

Dan heard her words, though they seemed a little distant simply because he was so much focused on what he was feeling. His head was spinning with it. Do this. Do that. In the programme people seemed to be keen to tell him what he should do, and part of him agreed, but then, he wasn't sure which part of him that was. And he just found himself more and more confused. He put his head in his hands, took a deep breath and blew the air out through his fingers. He drew his fingers down over his mouth and opened his eyes.

'I feel like I'm sitting here and I'm not sitting here.' He still had his fingers on his chin and the words came out indistinct. Jeannie found it hard to hear what he had said, so she repeated back what he said.

'Sorry, not sure that I caught that, sitting here but not sitting here?'

'Yeah. Like part of me is here but part of me isn't.' Dan stopped. 'No, that doesn't sound right. More all of me is here and all of me isn't.' He took another deep breath and breathed out deeply. 'This is madness.'

'Feels like madness.'

Dan nodded. He opened his mouth to speak, and closed it again. He was going to say 'yes' but somehow he kept quiet.

'Something hard to say?' Jeannie wanted to acknowledge what she had observed, and was curious what was being communicated to her.

The person-centred counsellor is seeking to be fully present themselves and is also seeking to respond to the whole person before them. Communication from the client is not only through words spoken. Dan has just communicated a struggle to say something and a process whereby what was about to be said was blocked. This happens for a reason. Jeannie isn't wanting to analyse it, but she has shown awareness of, and empathy towards, the process that has just occurred.

Dan nodded and stayed silent. He breathed in deep again and blew the air out. He really did feel anxious again, and his arms felt a little numb as well, his head slightly buzzy, a bit floaty and indistinct. He hated that word. And he hated the thought of applying it to himself. He'd always hated it.

Jeannie continued to sense the presence of the struggle within Dan. It was somehow very tangible. He may not have been speaking about it, but he was certainly communicating it through his manner, expression and body language. A couple more times he had looked as if he was about to say something, but seemed to pull back. 'It's really hard to say.'

He nodded. 'I hate it.'

'Hate it?'

'Yeah.'

Jeannie nodded slightly and tightened her lips, and then suddenly felt that her facial response was in a way mirroring Dan's tightening and blocking what he was struggling to say. 'Makes my lips go tight as well.'

Dan smiled, it was a weak smile, but it shifted his facial expression. 'Yeah. It's the thought of being, or of going, mad.' Dan closed his eyes and shook his head.

'You hate that thought . . .'

Dan stared towards the wall beside Jeannie and his expression somehow stopped her finishing her sentence.

'I was told I was mad. A long, long time ago. Well, quite a few times since as well, but I can remember my father standing there, it was after Billy, you know, standing there in the kitchen, drunk of course, looking down at me. I felt so small. And his voice, slurring but heavy and full of, I don't know, just felt like I was shit to him. Telling me that I was fucking, fucking mad. That's what he said. Told me I would die if I kept on the way I was. But he kept on at me, saying I was mad. I remember eventually running out of the room and upstairs in tears, and crying for, I don't know, must have been for ages.' Dan stopped and continued to stare at the wall, almost as if he was watching the events on a screen when in fact he was reliving them in his head.

'Felt so small, like shit, told you were mad and that you would die.'

'Yeah, and he said it was what I deserved. I remember that bit as well. "You'll fucking die and it'll be what you fucking deserve." '

Dan looked across to Jeannie. To Jeannie he suddenly looked very small and like a little boy. He's really connected, she thought, and maybe he really is that little boy in the room at this moment. She sought to empathise with this possibility.

'He's told you that you deserved to die.'

'I don't want to die, but I'm going to die. He told me. But I don't want to. I'm scared. I don't want to die. I don't. I really don't.' Dan's voice had changed. Jeannie really was talking to a very frightened, very hurt little boy.

'No, you don't want to die.'

'No, I don't, but he said I would. But I don't want to, I don't want to. Please, don't let me die.'

'I won't let you die.' Jeannie responded, seeking to offer the child within Dan some feeling of reassurance, recognising that maybe this was the first time he had been offered this.

'You won't?'

'No.'

'But he said . . .' Tears were trickling down Dan's cheeks.

'Yes, he said some nasty things to you, didn't he?'

'Yes, but you won't let me die.'

'No.'

Dan sighed. In that moment he changed, like he suddenly grew again. He burst into tears, uncontrollable tears, that went on and on. Jeannie thought about passing him a tissue but didn't, concerned that it might have conveyed some sort of suggestion that he should dry his eyes now. She wanted him to stay with what he was experiencing and expressing. Slowly the tears eased and then Jeannie passed him a tissue.

'Oooohhh.' Dan closed his eyes. That had been a shock and, oh, what feelings had rushed in on him. He really had felt so incredibly small and helpless and weak. He still felt weak, his legs, his arms. Like jelly, numb jelly but warm, not cold. 'That was me, wasn't it?' As he said it he felt how stupid that must sound.

'I think so.'

'Been carrying that around as well, haven't I?'

Jeannie nodded.

Another deep breath. 'I'd kind of forgotten that incident but it is now back with me, crystal clear. I really did relive something then, but it wasn't just in the past, was it? That part of me still exists, is with me now, isn't it?'

Jeannie nodded again. She didn't want to risk getting into some theoretical explanation, but wanted Dan to acknowledge to himself this part of who he was.

'A little boy, scared, terrified of dying. Terrified of dying.' He shook his head. 'And I spend most of the rest of my life doing things that could kill me. Bloody crazy. Jeannie, am I mad?'

As he spoke those last four words Dan's voice changed and so did the atmosphere in the room.

Here was one of those critical moments. She could empathise with Dan's need to know, she could tell him what she thought, she could try and straddle both, and she had no time to think about it because delay could convey that she wasn't coming from her authentic self. Yet to respond too quickly might be interpreted as being empty reassurance.

'No, Dan, I do not think you are mad. You have experienced a lot of hurt though and sometimes it feels like it to you.'

'Yeah, it does, but it's good to hear that you don't think I'm mad. And the way you spoke to me just now. Me? I mean that part of me. Well, not just a part of me, it really did feel like it was to me, telling me that you wouldn't let me die, that just swept through me, like a strong but warm, gentle breeze, I so needed to hear that, Jeannie. And I know as well that we all have to die, and you can't stop that, but it was the sense that someone out there cared enough to say what you said.'

'Yes, as an adult you know that I can't stop you dying one day, but that very hurt part of you needed to know that someone cared.'

Dan nodded. 'I don't think it was just that part of me; it affected all of me hearing what you were saying. It really has affected me. I don't know what I'm feeling now, sitting here, I've never been here before.' He stopped and thought for a while; Jeannie did not disturb his process. 'I don't think I've used this word for a long time, no, I did, in those earlier sessions when I felt so calm. But I feel somehow more at peace with myself. Yeah. Maybe some of the chaos has dissolved this evening. I hope so, Jeannie, I really hope so. The chaos will kill me if I don't change it.'

Feeling cared for has had a huge impact on Dan, challenging something deep inside himself. She offered unconditional positive regard towards the hurt, childlike part of Dan, spoke directly to it, reassuring it, offering it something that perhaps it never felt it really experienced, or if it did it was lost in the overwhelming reactions of his father to him.

Jeannie has also offered him reassurance, to Dan as the adult, that he is not mad. The latter could be regarded as the introduction of an external locus of evaluation, and arguably the client needs to eventually be able to trust their own self-belief that they are not mad. However, this is still a relatively early stage in the therapeutic relationship, and at present supporting Dan, reassuring Dan, is maybe what is most appropriate. As he frees himself from his 'conditions of worth' he will be more able to trust his own perceptions. At the moment he is confused and an outside voice saying in effect, 'It's OK, you're OK, keep with it, I'm here with you', has huge therapeutic value and is essentially a very human, person-to-person response.

The room went very quiet, very, very quiet. Jeannie looked at Dan, and he looked back at her. There was no need for words. They hung there, flashing above their heads and in their heads and hearts. Yes, she thought, the chaos will kill you if you don't change it. It's been trying to all your life.

Dan knew that Jeannie had appreciated the significance of what he had just heard himself say, and he was still taking it in himself. It summed him up, everything up: that was what it felt like, that he had embraced chaos as his normal; he had killed out the possibility of anything else. Shit, he thought, I hadn't thought of that before.

'Part of me died a long time ago; I killed part of myself when I chose chaos, when I chose to punish myself, when I chose to use, right the way through. But that part that was dead, I think it's coming to life again. I don't think it was really killed. You've breathed fresh life into me this session.' His eyes had opened a little more and a look of amazement had spread across his face.

'Coming back to life.'

'Yeah, something in me is coming back to life, and I need that part of me, need it to stop the chaos. I don't really understand it, not really, but something is happening, stirring inside me, and it feels good. It does feel good. I think I am experiencing it without the chaotic me telling me it isn't normal. That feels . . .' He took a deep breath and blew the air out slowly once more. 'That feels so good.'

'So good, yeah?'

'Yeah. I want to just stay with it.' Dan sat quietly for a few minutes, holding what he was feeling. Yes, something is different. He couldn't explain any of it, and somehow he didn't feel he really wanted to or needed to. It just felt good.

The session continued for the last few minutes with Dan saying how much he had to go away and think about, and how different he still felt, and how he hoped it would last but how he also realised that his 'chaotic me', the words he used, maybe hadn't completely gone. Jeannie empathised with this. It made her think of Mearns' theory of 'configurations of self', and that in effect Dan had identified a 'chaotic me' configuration of self.

Mearns suggests that 'the self is comprised of a number of "parts" or "configurations" interrelating like a family, with an individual variety of dynamics. When the interrelationship of configurations changes, it is not that we are left with something entirely new: we have the same "parts" as before, but some which may have been subservient before are stronger, others which were judged adversely are accepted, some which were in self-negating conflict have come to respect each other, and overall the parts have achieved constructive integration with the energy release which arises from such fusion' (Mearns and Thorne, 1999, pp.147–8). In this instance it is likely that Dan's 'chaotic me' configuration has been dominant for some time and will need to become subservient to either a currently weaker configuration that gains strength, or a new configuration that emerges as a result of the therapeutic process and developments within Dan's lifestyle.

Session 10

Dan arrived on time and started by explaining to Jeannie that he had had a difficult time returning to work now that the day programme had ended for him.
He had already talked it through with his keyworker but he also realised that
he needed time to talk about how he felt. It had felt safe being in the programme, and it had given him a lot to think about. It had been really stimulating, but back at work again, the monotony of his job had really struck home to
him. He realised he didn't like it and wanted to do something else, but didn't
know what. The first part of the session was therefore given over to him exploring options and wondering what he could do. He realised that he probably
needed more qualifications and so one option was to get himself along to the
local college of technology and check out what options there were.

'It's having a sense of wanting to move on and do something with my life, you
know. I'm going nowhere where I am, and I know it.'

'Mhmmm. Wanting to do something more fulfilling and feeling that otherwise
you are going nowhere.'

'Yeah. I just need something more. I guess that change is in the air at the moment
for me. I've also started reducing the methadone, very gradually, but I've made
the first drop and feel OK so far, little bit more on edge than usual the first day or
two, but now I'm feeling OK. I'm a bit apprehensive though, particularly as I'm
still off the alcohol. Don't want to push it, but I also want to get clean.'

'So, a little apprehensive but determined to reduce. Big step for you.'

'Sure is. But I'm taking it slowly. And I know if I need to stop reducing and stabilise that's OK. But I know it won't be easy, and I'm also a bit apprehensive
about what I will feel, you know, I mean not just the chemical reaction from
withdrawing, but what I may feel. I mean, I've experienced a lot here, and it
makes me wonder what else I'll feel and whether I can hold it together. It's
like stepping into the unknown here, and I'm really not sure what lies ahead.
But I need a focus, I need to be doing something constructive with my life as
part of all of this.'

Dan looked a mixture of determination and uncertainty. Jeannie responded to
this as she felt it was in tune with what he had just been saying. 'I see an air of
determination and uncertainty in you.'

Dan took a deep breath and let those words sink in. As he did so, another word
came into his mind. 'I need some stillness as well, time to just be, but I'm
afraid that feelings and memories will overwhelm me.'

'Mhmmm.'

Dan continued. 'I keep thinking back to some of the things that have happened in
our sessions, but the last session really stands out for me. The stuff about being
chaotic. Yeah, there is a "chaotic me". It has been with me for so long, as long
as I can remember. But it got me thinking, you know, because there's other
parts of me as well, you know?'

'Like we talked about last week towards the end of the session?'

'Yeah, not just "chaotic me"; I mean, a lot of my chaos has been linked to drug use, but it's more than that. So there's a "me the addict" which drives me to use and thrives on the experience, the thrill, the risk, the everything that goes with it, and it likes chaos as well. I started calling "chaotic me" a new name, "captain chaos", seems to sum it up. Kind of made me smile at it. Guess sometimes it's easier to laugh at yourself, otherwise I guess you'd cry. For all the excitement and craziness, "captain chaos" is really a sad figure, tragic.'

'So, "chaotic me" is "captain chaos" who's sad and tragic, yeah, and there's an "addict me".'

'Yeah, and they kind of go around together, you know?'

'Close relationship, yeah?'

'Buddies. Feels like "addict me" is a kind of dealer, dealing out what I need to nourish "captain chaos".'

'So "addict me" supplies "captain chaos"?'

'Yeah, every time. And I need to be more than either of these two; they are taking me nowhere and I've got to leave them behind somehow, ditch them, lose them, fucking waste them. They're no good to me, Jeannie, but I don't know what I'm trying to replace them with. I feel lost, alone, very small sometimes, like everything is so much bigger than I am. Yeah, there's a "little boy lost", isn't there, and he's around at the moment. I think I spend a lot of time being him at the moment, particularly since stopping using and I suppose he's become more present since I talked to you about Billy and about my father, how he reacted. Made me connect with him more, but he's not strong enough to deal with "addict me" and "captain chaos".'

'"Little boy lost" isn't strong enough . . .'

Dan shook his head. 'And it's scary. I feel so lost, you know, so unsure, and yet there is a determination in me as well. They nearly killed that little boy in me, and in a way I sort of want him to stay a little boy, but I also want him to grow up too. Like I wonder if that's what I really need, to grow up.'

'Guess I'm wondering what you mean by "grow up"?'

'Just be normal, that's who I want to be, just be normal.'

Jeannie listened to Dan and wondered whether this was the configuration that needed to emerge, to develop. She guessed there would always be a part of him like the little boy, but perhaps he could develop a sense of self that in a sense was able to care for that little boy part of himself. Oh-oh, she thought, I'm running away with notions here. Where's Dan at? Wanting to just be normal.

'So, just be normal, is that another part of you?'

Dan grinned. 'Yeah, I guess so. Yeah, "just be normal", yeah, that's what I want to be, but somehow I don't think I know who he is, you know? I mean, who is he, what is he? He's the guy I want to be; maybe he's the guy to stand up to "captain chaos" and "the addict".'

'You've changed the name, "addict me" becomes "the addict"?'

'Yeah I did, kind of sounds right somehow, more stark, easier to hate.'

'You hate "the addict"?'

'We all hate "the addict", all the parts of me hate "the addict". Even "captain chaos" hates "the addict". But "little boy lost", you know, I nearly said "little boy blue", and sounds right as well, 'cos he's sad and blue. Yeah, "little boy blue" is afraid of "the addict". He tried to kill him with drugs. Kept him silent, stopped him coming out to play, "captain chaos" took over and they were me, together, for a long time. I mean, I guess I wasn't just them, but they kind of, well, were me in so many ways. "Captain chaos" and "the addict", what a bloody horrible combination.'

'Don't think much of them then?' Jeannie knew she was understating. She probably was stepping out of being purely person-centred, but she couldn't help herself; she kind of felt she wanted to provoke a strong reaction.

'No I fucking don't. Fucked up my life for years, bastards. I could do without them, but they're around, waiting their chance. But I'm not going to give it to them. They make me so fucking angry.' Dan tightened his fists as he spoke this last sentence. He was angry; he really was angry.

Jeannie wasn't sure which part was present and carrying the anger. 'Where's the anger focused in you, Dan? Who's got the anger?'

'Fuck, I don't know.' He stopped and tried to feel where the anger was. 'Feels like it's a part of the me that I am. That doesn't make much sense. It isn't "just be normal", he's kind of wanting a quiet life, but then I guess maybe he needs to get angry sometimes. Can I have a part within a part?'

'Why not, you know what it feels like.'

'Well, this "angry me" is part of "just be normal", then. Yeah, that's where he is and where he needs to be. "Just be normal" wants a quiet life but wants to punch "captain chaos" 's lights out.'

The idea that a configuration could actually contain within it other parts is an interesting notion, and while it adds to the complexity, perhaps it is not unreasonable to hypothesise this possibility. The existence of what we might therefore term 'sub-configurations' implies that there is a kind of generational component to the family of configurations in the sense that they may exist at different levels.

'The "angry me" part of "just be normal" has a lot of anger to express and wants to point it at "captain chaos".'

'And "the addict". Yeah, I feel a real split, a real divide. Maybe that's not healthy, but that's how it is. And in the middle of all this is this sense of feeling small and lost, "little boy blue".' Dan stopped. 'You know, and this will sound weird, shit it's all fucking weird, but "little boy blue", you know, I think he's more important than I had thought. He's kind of strong in some way because he's kind of real? Am I making sense here?' Dan stopped to think for a moment. 'Let me just think about this.' 'The addict' was his drug-using self, OK, he could see that, and he was strong, but at the moment he, Dan, couldn't identify with him very strongly, the same with 'captain chaos'. 'You know, the bits that are most present for me at the moment are the "angry me" bit of "just be normal" and "little boy blue". I'm angry at parts of myself, and I'm feeling sad about it all, but lost when I look out into the world and try to work out where I'm going.' Dan took a deep breath. 'We've really taken off into all of this; it seems to be helping me make sense of me. It's confusing too, well, more complex than confusing, but it's like I've got a kind of map of myself and it's like there are symbols on the map representing parts of me, and I am beginning to find out what each of these symbols means. Each is a part with feelings and behaviours. Take "the addict": he just wants what he wants and to hell with what effect it has on anyone. He's mean. He doesn't give a shit about anything, so long as he gets what he wants. I want to get rid of him, but somehow he's part of me. I wish he was dead, but he's alive.'

'So you'd like to get rid of "the addict", yeah, kill him off, but you can't. He goes out and gets what he wants and to hell with the effect it has on anyone.'

'Yeah, he gets what he wants.' Dan stopped and thought about it. 'But has he only got to get drugs? I mean, OK, he's a problem, or he has been, but has he got to get drugs? Could he learn to get something else?'

'Could "the addict" find some other purpose, you mean?'

'Yeah, but "captain chaos" wouldn't like that. He'd die without the drugs.' Dan stopped again. 'You know, I thought "the addict" was the dealer, feeding "captain chaos", but I'm beginning to feel it's the other way around. It's the chaos in me that found the drugs and used them to perpetuate the chaos. It wasn't the drugs that created the chaos in my head, in my life; it was already there from my crap childhood.' He paused. 'Yeah, I've got it back to front, yeah.' He paused again. 'Yeah, this is really helpful.'

Jeannie nodded; she didn't want to obstruct or divert Dan's train of thought.

'So, I already learn chaos, yeah, and then I start using to, what I thought, get away from it, at least in my head, but it adds to it. Shit. It's like "captain chaos" created "the addict" so he could grow and get more powerful. Oh yeah, I can see now what I need to do, Jeannie, it's becoming clear. It's like I've got to turn "the addict" away from serving the needs of "captain chaos".'

'Turn him away and towards . . . ?'

'Towards . . .' Dan thought about it. What did he want to get for himself? What did he need the one-pointedness of 'the addict' for? Yes. It was like a light bulb coming on in his head. 'Yes, that's it. Yes. I need to turn "the addict" towards just being normal. That's the real battle, between "captain chaos" and "just be normal". I need "the addict" to switch allegiance.' A large grin broke out on Dan's face. 'Oh this is going to sound weird, man, oh geez. You know what I just thought? No, this is too crazy.' He grinned again.

'Go on, you can't not tell me after that build up!' Jeannie empathised with what she felt was the spirit of the moment.

'It's like turning Darth Vader from the dark side!' At which point Dan broke into laughter, and Jeannie found herself unable to control a grin that took over her face.

'Oh yeah? And who's Luke Skywalker in all of this?' Jeannie's reaction was totally spontaneous, no thought, just came out.

Dan went suddenly quiet. Oh shit, he thought, oh this isn't a joke. ' "Little boy blue." ' As he said it he suddenly felt a rush of emotion and his eyes watered. He rubbed his eyes and swallowed. 'Gee,' he said letting out a deep breath, 'that really touched me. I had the image in my mind in the film, which one, the first one, *Phantom Menace*, when as a little boy he has to leave his mother to go off with the Jedi, that moment when he runs back to her.' Dan could feel the emotion rising inside of himself, sadness, loneliness, smallness, all rushing in on him at once. He closed his eyes. He could feel the tears welling up again. 'I cried when I watched that part of the film. Something in me identified with him and now I know which part.'

Jeannie nodded, aware of how suddenly the atmosphere had changed from humour to a seriousness that made the atmosphere feel absolutely electric.

' "Little boy blue." '

Dan nodded, and swallowed. 'And "little boy blue" at some point has to face and turn "the addict" and destroy "captain chaos". And that feels awesome, and that feels right, and that's fucking scary. And I don't know what that means, but it somehow feels to me like it makes a lot of sense. The part of me that feels small and alone and scared has got to be encouraged to grow, to become strong, to become . . .' He stopped, trying to figure out what else he needed to become. 'I need to become what "little boy blue" had the potential to become, but he lost it to "captain chaos".' Dan stopped again. It had been a weird session; he had talked in ways that he hadn't expected, but he somehow felt a direction, a purpose, even though it was all tangled up in these strange ideas about having different bits. 'I need to become the me that I am, not be the me that I became.'

Jeannie reflected this back; she wanted Dan to hear it as he had said it so he could confirm if that really was what he meant. She spoke in the first person to add to the immediacy.

'I need to become the me that I am, not be the me that I became.'

Dan listened to his words being repeated back. Yes, he thought, but the 'I am' that is my potential, that I must reach for, that I must grow towards. He nodded. 'Yes, I can relate to that. And by the "me that I am" I think I mean the me that I feel now, here, in this moment. The me that isn't being dominated by chaos, the me that wants a normal life. The me that wants to grow up and have a normal life. Dammit, that's what I want, to grow up and have a normal life. That's it. That's it in a nutshell.'

'You sound like you have really connected with that wanting to grow up and live a normal life.'

'Yeah, I have, it feels more present in me somehow. I'm not sure quite how all we have talked about has done it, but each time, I'm going home with more determination.' He looked at the clock, not many minutes left.

'That's counselling, particularly the way I work, I guess. We really have ranged across all kinds of things, and I guess I have a sense that you already knew you wanted to live a normal life, but maybe it has become more affirmed within you, but the bit about wanting to grow up seems new somehow?' Jeannie was trying to sum up and also express her own perception of what the session had resulted in.

'The growing up bit is new, and I know what part of me I need to encourage to grow up and be strong. I need to care for a part of me that got hurt a long time ago, that is still very sensitive. I need to take care of myself, don't I? I mean really take care of myself. Part of me is precious; I need to really care for it, for me. I get lost in the words sometimes, it, me. It's me I need to care for. Healthy choices, Jeannie, I need to make healthy choices, and I need to go.'

The session drew to a close and they confirmed the appointment the following week.

Points for discussion

- How has reading these two sessions left you feeling, and what thoughts are in your head?
- How would you assess Jeannie's work with Dan in these two sessions from the perspective of person-centred theory?
- Where might you have made different responses to Dan during the course of these two sessions?
- Was the 'Luke Skywalker' question appropriate? What do you think was happening in that interaction?
- Discuss the notion of 'configurations of self'. What are your views on this theoretical explanation for human experiencing?
- Dan has ended up making some clear and powerful affirmations about himself. Which part of himself is speaking here?

Summary

Dan explores his developing sense of his 'normal' being all wrong, and of how scary that is. He talks of feeling split. He reconnects with memories of being told he was mad as a child and how difficult it is for him as an adult to talk about feeling mad. Jeannie engages with him both in a childlike state and as an adult, and offers him caring and reassurance which have a powerful effect on Dan. He recognises for himself that in embracing chaos he allowed another part of himself to almost die. The notion of Dan having different 'parts' within himself emerges and he names these and explores them and their inter-relationships. He draws a parallel between his process and the theme of the *Star Wars* movies, bringing him to a very poignant moment of acknowledging what he needs to do.

CHAPTER 8

Further 'parts' emerge and the metaphor of a jigsaw of self arises

Session 11

Dan arrived the following week and it had been quite a week for him. He began by telling Jeannie what had been going on.

'When I left here last week I really felt positive; I really had a sense of direction and a feel for myself that was different to anything I had experienced before. That stuff we talked about, the parts of me, that just made so much sense. It really helped and I talked to Gemma about it. She was intrigued as well, though I think a little confused at times. But for me, it just made sense. But what I ran into problems with was that while I know I need to grow up and all that, what I now realise I don't know is what that actually means, or at least, how I can kind of cope with it.'

Clients will use the time between sessions and this is so important and an indicator of the impact that the therapeutic experience is having on them.

Jeannie had listened carefully to what Dan had been saying, and she was struck by a sense of a kind of neediness which also made her think of that little boy part of him. Here he was, trying to make his way in an adult world, but a major part of himself was still that little boy. 'How to grow up and how to cope with, what, grown up things?' Jeannie wasn't too sure what Dan wanted to learn to cope with.

'Just doing adult things, I mean, well, stuff around the house. I can so easily just go and sit on my own and watch TV, or read a magazine or something, or play computer games, you know. And that annoys Gemma, and she has a go about something that needs doing and I find it really difficult to respond in a kind of helpful way.'

'So your response isn't very helpful. That's how it feels?'

'Yeah, I just feel that clearing out the junk from the garage or clearing up outside, or putting a shelf up, well, it's just, well, it's boring, isn't it?'

'So you are having difficulty tolerating doing things that are boring?'

'Yes, well, no, I mean, well, I'm not actually doing them.'

'So it's the thought of doing them?'

Dan thought about it. 'Yesterday, in the evening, it was quite warm and Gemma was outside and she needed some stuff put away. She asked me to do it, and I said I would, but later. But I didn't do it, just carried on with this computer game. Seem to have really got into them recently. So we ended up arguing about it, and, well, it really made me feel like going for a drink, you know? But I didn't and that was good. But I just seem to find reasons for not doing things that maybe I should do, or it would be normal to do, you know?'

'OK, let me check out that I've got this right. Gemma asked you to do something outside, you said yes but later, though you just carried on with the computer game, didn't do it, had an argument, felt like a drink, but didn't. And your sense is that you are finding reasons not to do things, normal things.'

'Yeah. I really can't seem to feel enthusiasm for stuff like that.'

'So it doesn't fire you with enthusiasm.'

'No. It's like I've been at work all day, get home, and just want to relax, just want to do what I want.'

'So it's about doing what you want to do?'

'Yeah, well, I suppose so.' Dan was suddenly aware that this now felt a little bit uncomfortable. 'Yeah, I guess that's how it is, but I also don't feel good about it as well.'

'Don't feel good about doing what you want to do?'

This response could be regarded as challenging. Yes, it has that effect and yet this is not the intention for Jeannie as a person-centred counsellor. She is simply voicing her empathic sense of what has been said by Dan, inviting further exploration. Yet the effect on Dan is that of being quite challenging and immediate. His body language reflects that it has made an impact even though he has only heard what he has already said.

Dan tightened his lips and drew a breath in through his teeth. 'I don't know. I feel mixed up. I want to be normal, but I want to do my own thing. They seem to be different, somehow, and I'm choosing what I want, and it's causing problems.'

'Choosing to do what you want causes problems with Gemma.'

'Yeah, but not just with Gemma, with me, too. I don't enjoy what I do so much. Or at least, I kind of do at the time but then afterwards that gets wiped out if we have an argument, and I feel angry but also guilty, though more angry than guilty.'

'Angry with? Guilty about?'

'Angry with Gemma for making me uncomfortable. Then angry with myself for not being able to do something that I know is normal, and then guilty about not doing it as well. And then the anger towards her comes back again, because I don't want to do what she wants me to do. She gets on my case, I react. It's getting really difficult. And yet I know I love her as well, but I'm just not helping myself. I feel stuck. I don't know how to get out of it.'

Jeannie was experiencing an overwhelming urge to ask Dan what he wanted to do, what he really wanted to do, yet she also wanted to empathise with him. She decided to focus on the latter, placing empathy first. 'You really love her, Dan . . .'

'I do.'

'. . . but you feel stuck and you don't know how to get out of it.'

'I don't. I wish I could motivate myself. I left here really fired up, but somehow I lost that motivation.'

Jeannie wondered whether it might be the methadone. But she also felt it was probably 'the addict'. It sounded like it was that 'I'm gonna do what I want to do' part of himself that was in control. Jeannie replied slowly, 'So, you have trouble holding on to the motivation.'

'Just can't seem to get a grip on myself, and it's crazy. I should be able to do this, but I can't, and it's getting between Gemma and me and I really don't want that.'

'No, I really do hear you say that, Dan; she's really important to you, isn't she?'

He nodded. 'Yes. It's me. I know it's me. It's my stupid habits from the past getting in the fucking way. And I'm so pissed off with myself really. I talk about her being on my case, but it's not her really. She's only asking reasonable things. It's me.'

'You really do blame yourself, Dan.'

Dan seems to have heard Jeannie in such a way as to think she is trying to indicate he is not all to blame. But he reacts to this by owning his need to blame himself, probably linked to his feelings of guilt from the past. His self-blame in the present is heightened by what he has experienced in the past and therefore his current feelings can become out of proportion to the present situation.

'But it is me. She's being reasonable, I'm not.' Dan closed his eyes; he was suddenly feeling very tired.

He might also be tired of feeling not heard if that is what he is sensing from Jeannie. He now switches to another focus.

'I get tired and I think it's the methadone, coming off it. I think it's making me more reactive but also more drained. I don't know, I think I need to talk to

Marie about it. I'm not sure if this is a reaction to reducing, which I'm still doing, or if it is something else.'

'Mhmmm. You want to make sense of what is happening, and why.'

'If it's the methadone, then OK, I have to accept that and just keep trying, I guess. But if it's me, I don't know. I spend a lot of time with those games now, a lot of time. It is worrying me though at the time I just lose myself in them.'

'Lose yourself? What parts do you lose, Dan?'

'Um, well, I guess I, er, I don't know.' He genuinely didn't know. He sat there, just totally absorbed, total concentration, nothing else troubled him and he didn't think about anything else. He felt strangely anxious. He hadn't expected such a direct question; at least, that was how it had felt. It left him on edge. 'Everything, I guess.'

'Everything?'

'Well, yes, why, do you think that it isn't everything?'

'So what part keeps you playing?'

Jeannie's got herself into a bit of a question and answer session which has left Dan struggling for words and ending up asking her a question. She has strayed from person-centred working. She has attempted to direct his focus to the parts that he loses, and Dan is not ready for this. Such a directive enquiry can feel quite invasive for a client. Had she just said 'Lose yourself?' then Dan would have been allowed to explore it in his own way and with his own chosen focus and emphasis. He then tries to free himself from this by asking Jeannie a direct question and she ignores it and asks another question herself. Dan will be left feeling anxious and uncertain. Momentarily he has lost his sense of safety in the relationship and his sense of being free to explore. But he recovers from this and moves on. Jeannie has lost her person-centred focus. It does not get raised in supervision because she is unaware of what she has done. Such instances are cases for taping sessions and reflecting on them later.

He thought about it. Well, these are adult games so it isn't the little boy in me. And I have to be focused, so it isn't about chaos. ' "The addict." He's keeping me there, and it is like an addiction, isn't it?' He thought a bit more and nodded his head. 'And it is threatening, well, causing chaos between me and Gemma. OK.' Dan thought again about what he needed to do. 'OK, so I have to break that addiction, do something else. You know, it is like an addiction; once I start it is hard to stop.'

'Hard?'

'Yes, well, I don't stop, do I? It is really like an addiction. I just ignore everything else and just have to keep going, even though it causes problems. So I mustn't start, must I? I mean, I need to not start playing those games, then I might choose something else. But then I have to tolerate that something else. Shit. It seemed so easy last week, making changes, moving on, growing up and stuff.

But it's bloody hard.' He blew out a long, deep breath.' 'Bloody hard, yeah.' He paused. 'So, I have to not start on those games, I have to already start doing something else. Hmmm.'

'You need to change your routine around in the evenings, yeah.'

'Yeah, I do, I have to. It'll be a disaster if I don't. It'll be . . .' Dan realised what he was about to say, and it struck him with a lot of force. He looked at Jeannie. 'It'll cause a lot of chaos if I don't. Captain fucking chaos. Shit. It's a bloody battle, isn't it, with an invisible enemy inside myself.'

'Who only appears through your behaviours and attitudes.'

Jeannie hasn't empathised; she has reacted by adding detail to what Dan has said. In a sense she has stepped out of his frame of reference although what she has said is also true.

'Yeah.' Dan had a look of resignation on his face. 'Yeah, invisible except when he appears and then it's too late. It's happening. I've got to head him off, stop him. I've got to. Or else . . .' Dan knew what it would mean: he'd lose everything, he'd put himself at risk of losing Gemma and then, well, relapsing on everything. He went cold at the thought of it and knew he couldn't face that. 'I can't risk losing her, Jeannie, I can't. I've got to make real changes, and really make them, not just talk about them.'

'Time for action, yeah, time for real change.'

'I've no choice any more. It's like everything is becoming sharper and narrower, like my choices are becoming clearer but I still have to make them. It's all coming down to whether I make choices that lead to chaos, or those that do not. It's as simple as that. Yet it isn't simple, is it? I mean, playing computer games feels like a choice that avoids chaos, but it isn't really. It causes it. Have I got to question everything I do?'

Jeannie instinctively nodded.

'Oh shit.' He paused, then continued. 'You're right, of course, but still, oh shit!'

Dan found it hard to imagine exactly what this meant, though he had a sense that he really was going to have to undergo fundamental changes in attitude, and yet he couldn't see how he could impose them on himself. That felt like, well, mission impossible. And yet he knew that the person he was at the moment needed to be different.

In order to generate a sustainable change in behaviour, there is a need for inner change as well. This is slowly sinking in for Dan. He cannot conceive of himself other than who he is, and yet he knows he needs to change. Without a doubt, clients are courageous adventurers, pioneers, pursuing a path of personal re-creation, and often without really knowing what kind of person will emerge from the therapeutic process.

'It's strange, but over the last couple of weeks or so I really have become more aware of the different parts of myself, and I can kind of sense myself moving between them, though often not at the time. Only in retrospect. But not every day because I kind of forget about thinking about it as well.'

'Mhmmm.'

'And yet, fundamentally, I still feel lost in myself, and afraid that chaos will regain control once more. I keep talking about it but it doesn't take away the sense that it could happen, you know?'

'Yeah, talking doesn't change what you feel about chaos.' No, thought Jeannie, that wasn't what he said; why did I go and respond like that? 'Sorry, you didn't say that, did you? It's the sense that it could still happen that talking isn't taking away.'

Jeannie's comment was not an empathic one, but she noticed it and corrected herself, which could actually have a powerful therapeutic effect in that it shows Dan that Jeannie isn't only listening to him, but also to what she is saying in response.

'Yeah, it could. I feel quite wobbly as I think about it, and it is linked to feeling small. That's really powerful, you know, and yet here I am, fifteen stone, not enormous but pretty big, and yet I feel really small.'

'You sound surprised by that?'

'I don't know, I suppose I am. But it is weird. I can feel myself, my skin, the edge of me.' He waved his hands as he said it to try and indicate his physical edge. 'And yet sometimes I feel as though I don't really fill my own body, my own space. Like I'm lost somewhere inside me, somewhere.'

'Mhmmm, feeling lost inside yourself, and not sure quite where you are?'

'And I . . . , ooh that's weird.'

Jeannie raised her brows slightly, acknowledging Dan's comment.

'It's like I feel too small sometimes to drive this big body.'

'Mhmmm, so you feel your body is kind of too big for you to drive around in?'

'Yeah, but drive sounds wrong, doesn't it, maybe to just move around, to make it do and go where I want it to go.'

'So too big for you to move around and make it do and go where you want.'

'That sounds more like it, hearing you say it, yeah. Like I only come up to here in myself.' Dan held his hand just above his solar plexus. 'I don't feel like I come above here when I'm feeling lost. I kind of shrink, but shrink downwards.'

'So feeling is linked to shrinking inside yourself.'

'But I don't feel shrinking inside myself; it's me that's shrinking. I just feel small, alone, and, yeah, it's like people don't see me, like I'm kind of hidden, like they talk over me.'

'Do you mean talk to your big body but not to the little person you become inside?'

Dan thought for a moment. That sort of sounded right, but he wasn't sure. 'Ye-es, and yet, I don't know.' He shook his head. 'That's kind of right but it isn't. It's really difficult to describe, and yet when I am feeling it, it is so real.'

Dan sat and thought about it some more. He closed his eyes and imagined himself shrinking down, and he found that he could, but immediately he started feeling all the discomfort that came with it. He could feel himself becoming anxious, feeling lost, more lost than he was talking about just before. He felt very shy all of a sudden and didn't feel he could say anything. It was really uncomfortable now; he wanted to move but he felt unable to, like he couldn't make his body move and he felt afraid that he would look awkward.

Jeannie had felt a shift in her perspective as she observed Dan sitting thinking. She sensed something had happened and so she asked him if there was anything he wanted to say, speaking softly. And then added, 'Can you tell me what it is like?'

Dan tightened his lips. He opened his mouth, but nothing came out and he closed it again. This happened two more times. Jeannie smiled and Dan noticed it; it was a warm smile and it made him feel somehow more safe. He tried again; this time he was able to speak. 'I'm afraid, I'm really afraid. I can't seem to . . . to do anything. I feel stuck, like I'm in a thick fog and I can't clear it or move. It's all around me, and it's in my head too. I'm afraid, I can't seem to do anything. It's like I'm kind of frozen but I'm not cold.'

'You feel frozen but not cold, stuck in a thick fog, can't move, and it makes you very afraid.'

Dan nodded. 'Can't move, want to move, but can't move. This fog, it's weird, it's a weird colour.'

'Weird colour?'

'Yeah, like it's kind of greenish, sort of, but not all the time. It stops me from moving and from seeing where I'm going.'

Jeannie realised that she was talking to the small part in Dan, of the small part that at this moment was Dan. She felt that what he was saying was important, but she wasn't sure what he wanted her to understand. She tried to encourage him to say more. 'The greenish fog, it's sort of holding you back?'

'Yes. Can't seem to think clearly, can't seem to find my direction in this fog.'

'The fog stops you thinking or seeing clearly.'

'Yes. "The addict" makes it happen.'

Jeannie was sure that her expression must have conveyed surprise. ' "The addict"?'

'Yes, he makes me drink the fog, says I have to have it. I think he's right, it's safe in the fog, but I also feel stuck as well.'

' "The addict" makes you drink the fog, and it's a safe fog and a stuck-in-it fog.'

'Want to get out of the fog but I'm afraid what I will see.'

Jeannie nodded. 'Mhmmm, so you want to get out but that's scary because of what you might then see.' Jeannie had realised what the fog represented. But she wasn't there to make the connection. At some level Dan knew too. She continued to listen.

'I feel very hurt. I feel very sad. I want to get out. Please help me get out.'

'I will help you get out, Dan.'

'Thank you. But my friends call me Danny.'

'OK, Danny.'

'Sometimes the fog is thinner, sometimes thicker. It's thicker in the mornings and then gets thinner later.'

That was all Jeannie needed to confirm her suspicions. It's the bloody methadone: it's green, it's putting a fog around this part of Dan, which she assumed was the configuration they had identified in the last session as 'little boy blue'. Maybe I should check this out, though, she asked herself. Check out assumptions. Could be that Danny is another part, but he sounded so much like how she would expect 'little boy blue' to be.

'Danny, I hear what you say about the fog thinning later in the day. Can I check something out with you? Is Danny also "little boy blue"?'

'Yes.'

'And "the addict" makes you drink the fog each day and makes you feel lost and stuck?'

'Yes. I wish he'd stop. But I'm glad he doesn't as well 'cos I'm afraid of what it will be like without the fog. When it thins I start to feel very sad and lonely and shy, and I don't like it.'

'No, Danny, you don't like it getting thinner but part of you would like the fog to go away as well.' Jeannie could feel her concentration levels set to maximum as she sought to stay closely with what Dan, no, Danny, was saying to her.

'When it gets thinner I do other things, play games, "the addict" tells me to. I like the games, and then I sleep, and then I have to drink more fog.'

Throughout the conversation Dan was Danny; he wasn't somehow watching and listening as an adult to what this part of himself was saying. Dan was Danny: that was the only reality, the only sense of self that was present within Dan's body.

This is an important point. Mearns' 'configurations of self' (Mearns and Thorne, 2000) are distinct from what have become termed 'dissociated parts', emerging within what is termed 'dissociative process' (Warner, 2000, 2002). The latter arise more from traumatic events such as sexual abuse, often in early childhood, while 'configurations' are regarded as normal features within the structure of self, developing in response to the intense symbolisation of experiences that can take place particularly during formative years but not exclusively so. Whereas dissociated parts can assume their own identity and become quite independent and unaware of other dissociated parts, configurations tend to be more of a family, bound together in relationship and with a continuity of awareness flowing through and between them.

'We have to drink more fog, it keeps us aliiiiive, it keeps us saaaaaafe, it keeps us commmmmfortable.' The voice had changed and it was not a nice voice to listen to. It spoke slowly and lingered over some of the words. 'We need it and we must have it. But they are taking it awaaaay from us, and we don't like it. No, we don't like it. We must have it.'

'The addict' thought Jeannie. 'Where is "little boy blue"?'

'Don't worry about him, I'll keep him saaaafe, keep him quiiiiet.'

'You really do want to keep topping up with the methadone, don't you?'

'Yes, and we will, and we won't let them take it away from us.'

'You must be very afraid of having it taken away?'

'No, we're not afraid, we're not afraid because they won't take it away.'

'But they are, aren't they?'

'We'll see. I really do need the methadone, you know, it keeps me sane, keeps me together, but I want to be clear and clean and I want to get in control again.'

'I know, Dan, I know.'

'But, well, that was spooky just then but that was me, they were me, that's what I feel.'

'Yes, they're parts of you, Dan, and they are in conflict and have been for a long time.'

'Yes, but "the addict" isn't going to win; what just happened has helped me again to see what I need to do. It's the methadone, isn't it, that's stopping me grow now. Throughout my life I've used substances and they have held me back, stopped me feeling things, put me in a fog a lot of the time; now it is thinner, and it is going to get thinner and, yes, I'm shit-scared as to how I'll be without it, but I'm going to succeed. But I've got to break "the addict" in me if I'm to be normal.'

'That's what you feel, to succeed you must break the addict in you.'

'And it helps to think of it as a part of me, but in a sense it is so much of me, it has been so much of my life.' Dan blew out a deep breath. 'This process is absolutely amazing, Jeannie, I go away with so much to think about, though it does fade a bit during the week, and I still haven't broken the addictive part of me, yet. But I have another week to go and battle with it.'

Jeannie had noticed the time; the session had almost overrun. She had been so engrossed with what was happening she had lost all sense of time. She mentioned it to Dan, and the session drew to a close. Jeannie checked that Dan felt sufficiently together to head off, and he said that he felt that he was, and he departed.

Session 12

Jeannie glanced at the clock; it was time for Dan to arrive, and she strolled out to the waiting area to see if he had arrived. He wasn't there, so she returned to the counselling room. She had spent a lot of time reflecting on that last session. The parts of Dan that had emerged seemed very distinct and she was left wondering whether they really were 'configuration with the Self', or whether they were 'dissociated parts'. They just had such profound, independent identities. She realised that she wasn't sure, but she knew that it depended on their origin.

Dan had been traumatised by the death of Billy, and yet he was older than she would have expected for dissociation, although she knew it was still possible. But that hadn't been the effect on Dan when he spoke about Billy's death. He had simply seemed like a very scared little boy, which added more fear to a little boy already experiencing this at home.

Her mind had then taken her to wonder about the impact of the chemicals on this kind of developmental process. Could drug use in some way induce a greater state of independence among the configurations? She simply did not know. Certainly, Dan had fragmentation and yet that just didn't feel like the right word for it. She knew she had a lot to talk through in supervision next time. Time and again her mind had kept coming back to wondering what the drugs might have done to affect the emergence of configurations during the developmental process.

So she sat, lost in her thoughts, and lost all track of time as well. Almost ten minutes had passed when she looked at the clock. She sat up with a jolt, got up and went to the waiting room. Dan was sitting, waiting. The receptionist was on the phone; presumably she hadn't been able to tell her Dan had arrived, or had forgot. Anyway, it wasn't her to blame; she shouldn't have drifted off into her thoughts. But she had, and that was another issue for supervision. Was it a reaction that would keep her distant from the impact of Dan, reducing the length of the session? She had drifted again. More supervision needed. She pushed the thoughts aside as they entered the counselling room.

'Hi Dan, sorry about causing you to wait. It was my fault; I was thinking about what has been happening in our sessions and I got lost in my thoughts.'

Jeannie had decided to be open about the reason for Dan's wait. She wanted to be open and transparent, and the delay had been the result of their relationship. She felt it was important to be open; she could speak about it in a relaxed manner and it meant that the session started with a genuine expression of authenticity.

'Oh, right.' Dan was somewhat taken aback. He had been sitting there, wondering what was happening, but had assumed that Jeannie must have been on the phone, or running late or something. It somehow affected him that she had been thinking about him, and about their sessions. He was curious now as to what she had been thinking about. 'So, what's your verdict then?'

Jeannie smiled. 'I was wondering about what impact your drug use over the years would have had on your development as a person, you know.' Oh no, she thought, now I've picked up on his verbal mannerism. 'And I don't have an answer.'

'I wonder that as well. Drugs have been such a big part of my life for so long. I mean, I guess I've been drug-affected so much that it is hard to really know who I am, and who I've been. But it's changing, slowly. I'm staying off the alcohol; in fact, I decided to start going to Alcoholics Anonymous. Just thought it might help a bit, you know, and, yeah, I've been a couple of times. After last session I just sensed that I needed all the help I could get. Alcohol got me back into the gear last time and I wanted to block that route, know what I mean?'

'Yes, that sounds like a very positive step, and I hope that it will help you. No one else can offer the 24/7 service that you can get through AA, with meetings, telephone help and sponsors, so if it works for you, go for it.'

'Thanks. It felt important. I had sort of thought about it before, but, well, something else I didn't get round to, you know? The addict in me getting in the way. But this feels good, feels positive, feels what I need to do.'

Jeannie felt a familiar thought arising in her head, something she had pondered on many times: how some people genuinely worked the AA programme and truly moved on in themselves, but others just switched addiction and seemed to get stuck going to meetings but without really moving on in themselves – the 'dry drunk' she thought they called it. Maybe, she thought, maybe Dan is turning 'the addict', and may not even be thinking of it in those terms. She kept her thoughts to herself.

This kind of insight is best discovered by the client. The counsellor, whether they are person-centred or not, who makes connections for clients and keeps getting ahead of them is a menace. Let the client grow at their own pace, and make their own connections as they develop their own fresh insight. An attempt to force growth does not create healthy plants and it probably doesn't create healthy people either.

'So, feels like a really good, positive decision, and what you need to do.'

'Yeah, I've only been twice, couldn't go, what do they say, ninety meetings in ninety days, Gemma'd go mad. But it has helped break the pattern of the computer games. I am doing other things now in the evenings, and I'm keeping away from them. So that feels good and it has made it easier at home. I've reduced the methadone again, and so far so good. I'm at 15 mls a day now. Going to hold that for a couple of weeks if I can and then review it with Marie and the doctor.'

'So, big changes. Something about the last session?'

'Yeah. Just found more determination from somewhere, don't know where. Just felt more ready to go for it, and found that I could. I'm not sure that I felt all that much different, but I just did it. I went to a meeting on the Friday evening, over at Alburton. And then another Sunday evening, this time at Chilham. Yeah, it felt good. Bit apprehensive both times, it's all new to me, but people were really friendly and they seemed genuinely pleased that I was there. Didn't speak at either of the meetings, just listened. Obviously, people were talking about alcohol and though I've used alcohol all my life, it was more the drugs that messed me up, I think. But there were similar stories, and the feelings people expressed, I just sat nodding my head. So many people feeling guilty, blaming themselves, feeling ashamed about things they've done. I know what that's like.' Dan shrugged. 'So, that's me, my name is Dan and I'm an alcoholic.'

'Do you believe that?'

'Actually no, I think of myself more in terms of addiction, "the addict", you know, but I realise that alcohol puts me at risk and I just felt that was where I needed to be.'

'Just curious that you didn't decide to go to Narcotics Anonymous (NA).'

'Don't know, just somehow felt that I wanted to focus on keeping off the alcohol.'

'Yeah, just wanted to keep that focus, keeping dry.'

Dan was aware as he had spoken that it wasn't just that. Hearing Jeannie repeat back the gist of what he had said he knew it wasn't the whole story. He felt anxious. He knew he had to be real with her, and with himself. What was the point if he wasn't? 'I have to be honest with you, that wasn't the only reason. I didn't want to hear about people using drugs, just feel that, I don't know, I've really got that out of my head at the moment and, well, I just thought that it wouldn't be a good idea, not at the moment.'

'Dan, I really appreciate you being open about that. I think it is a difficult decision and you have thought it through and decided what feels right for you. Yeah? You've trusted your instincts.'

'Yeah. I sort of thought you might have said I was crazy for avoiding NA.'

'You thought I would think you were crazy? No. I think you have made a choice based on what feels right for you. I support you in that.'

Jeannie has reassured Dan but also highlighted her valuing of his making his own decision and trusting his own instincts. In a sense, her comments flow towards Dan from an 'external locus of evaluation', but with the intention of encouraging him in trusting his own 'internal locus of evaluation'.

Dan felt a wave of ease pass through him. That felt good, he thought, he really hadn't been sure how Jeannie might react. And it was good to have her opinion, and good to feel trusted too. He took a deep breath. 'Thanks. We'll see, I may change, I don't know, but at the moment this feels right for me.'

'Mhmmm. Go for what feels right.'

'Yeah, got to get some order into my life. Get that chaos out of my head, forever.' Dan lifted his hands over his mouth, as if he was about to say something but had changed his mind. In fact, Dan was thinking about something that had just struck him. 'You know, that last session, and maybe the ones just before it, they weren't easy and I can't say I really understood what was going on a lot of the time, and I can't even remember a lot of it either, which is strange but then my memory's not too good, another effect of my drugs choices I guess, but ... well, I kind of feel I know myself better? Does that make sense?'

'Makes sense to me, though I'm curious what knowing yourself better means to you?'

Dan thought for a while. He found it hard to really get hold of exactly what he meant. He just sensed a difference. 'It's like ... well, the best image I can come up with is if you think of a jigsaw. Loads of pieces, all face down. It feels like

I've started to turn some of them over and can now begin to get a sense of how they may fit together. I don't know what the whole picture is, but I feel like I've started to begin to put it together. Does that makes sense?'

'It does,' Jeannie replied, congruently because it did make sense to her. 'You're getting to see what's on some of the pieces and finding how some of them fit together, finding parts of you and seeing how they fit together.'

'And it somehow makes me feel stronger, somehow more together, less in bits, although there are still lots of pieces.'

'Mhmmm, putting parts of yourself together makes you feel stronger?'

'Yeah, and I think that's what's happening, slowly, mind you, but I think that's what's happening. I'm beginning to put myself together.'

Jeannie smiled. 'That's great, must feel so good to feel that this is happening.'

Dan smiled as well. 'Yeah, but I know there is a long way to go, a long way to go.'

'Mhmmm. Lots of pieces, yeah?'

'Lots of pieces. And you know, I don't think some of them even fit in my picture.'

This is an important recognition and one that needs to be strongly empathised with. Dan is realising that parts of what make him who he is may not in reality fit in his final picture. He is acknowledging that he may need to reject parts of himself.

'Some are not part of your picture?'

'No. Some parts of me I think are pieces I've picked up from other people, people I've copied but who were full of shit, people I've looked up to and maybe shouldn't have, ideas and behaviours that seemed right at the time but were crap. I think there are a lot of pieces that won't fit in my final picture, and I've got to get rid of them, burn them, just get them out of the way 'cos they are going to get in the way, confuse me. I need to find them and get shot of them.'

'So you sound like you want to look for them so you can get shot of them?'

'I don't know if I want to look for them. I kind of imagine they'll be obviously not part of me as I build the picture. But I may need to look for them as well, but I guess I'll only know if I have to throw them away if they don't seem to fit, but I also need to be sure, don't I, that I throw the right ones away. Shit, hadn't thought of that. I've got to be careful here.'

'Yeah, slowly, slowly. Might not be easy to recognise which ones to keep and which ones to throw away.'

'So how can I be sure?'

'How can you be sure?'

Dan was feeling anxious now, he hadn't thought about this; in fact the whole idea of the jigsaw was something he was thinking through as he spoke, but it just seemed to make so much sense to describe what was happening to him. 'Well, I guess I don't really know. The only test I have is whether or not they fit onto what I have already pieced together. I haven't got a picture to follow. So I won't know, will I, until ... until more of the picture is created, which means until more of me comes together. So, take it slowly, take it carefully, but keep my focus on what I am building, not on what I am discarding? Is that right? That seems kind of logical but it also means I'm maybe hanging on to pieces that could end up confusing me, but they might turn out to be the pieces I need. Shit, this is complicated, and yet it isn't, is it? It's just doing a jigsaw. I'm just putting myself together, but I can choose which pieces I use.' Dan paused. He felt a sudden rush of energy and a quickening of his heartbeat. 'And which pieces I use will govern what the final picture looks like.'

'Yes.' Jeannie smiled. 'The pieces that you choose to fit together will govern what picture emerges.'

'And in terms of me,' Dan was speaking slowly as he was thinking and trying to grasp the implications of it all, 'so in terms of me, the choices I make now will govern what emerges in me, what, I guess, I'll finally look like.'

'Mhmmm. Your choices, yeah? Govern what you finally look like.'

Dan sat somewhat awestruck by all of this, and yet it just made so much sense. It was like a revelation to him. Yet at some level he knew it made sense. Yes, he could re-create himself, he had to work though what he wanted of himself. A thought struck him. 'But the bits that don't seem to fit now. The bits of me that get in the way of me becoming who I want to be, more normal, you know, less of the addict, less of the chaos, I mean, in a way they are part of me, right, so I guess . . .' Dan realised that he had confused himself. He stopped and thought about it.

Jeannie noted the confused look on Dan's face yet she also felt she wanted to leave him with space to reflect further on whatever he had been trying to say, to maybe clarify his thinking for himself rather than leaving him feeling he couldn't deal with what seemed to be so confusing to him.

Although Jeannie is making an assumption regarding Dan's confusion, she is basing it on what she perceives from his facial expression and the nature of what he had been saying before he stopped talking. She could have empathised with the confusion and thereby left Dan in the confused state or, as she has chosen, allow him his own space to find his own way through it without her emphasising the confusion that he is already perfectly well aware of.

'I guess it's the thought that I won't know which parts of me will be part of the final picture until it emerges more clearly, so I have to carry the, if you like, dodgy bits, with me, and they could threaten a lapse back into the old me.'

Jeannie nodded. 'Mhmmm, that's a real concern. If you hang on to the pieces, parts of yourself that don't seem to fit at the moment, will they end up putting you at risk of a relapse?'

'And I don't mean just on the alcohol or the drugs, but into old patterns of behaviour.'

'Yes, it's more than just the substances.'

Dan thought more. 'It feels scary, this. I feel I need to just get this together in my head. What I'm feeling here is that within me are different parts, represented by different pieces in a jigsaw. They are face down but I am turning them over, seeing what they are and deciding which I want to place into the final picture, the me that I am striving to become, the "normal" me that's grown away from, or out of, the drugs, the drinking, the chaos, the ... the everything that I've known for so long. And there are pieces, parts of me, that are new or developing which I want to include in that final picture. Like doing things without getting bored by them, studying, getting myself on in life and in work, taking more responsibility, being an adult, being less needy and demanding of others.'

'Mhmmm, quite a lot of pieces ...'

'Yes, but it all comes down to me growing up.' Dan stopped. He was back feeling small. ' "Little boy blue" has to grow up, he has to become what I want to be; I left him behind, that's the "I" ruled by "the addict" and "captain chaos". I became those two so much of my life.' Dan felt a sudden burst of anger within himself, and he was taken aback by the strength of it. 'I hate those bastards, they've fucked my life up, I don't want them around any more, they can both fuck off for all I care.'

'Fuck "the addict" and "captain chaos".'

Dan went silent. 'Yeah,' but his voice had changed and his tone had quietened, 'but I can't do that, they are parts of who I am and I may need them in some way, but I don't want to be ruled by them. So I have to be strong, I have to make changes. I have to,' he lost himself in his thought again, 'I have to start being true to another side of myself.'

'True to another side of yourself?' Jeannie wasn't sure precisely what Dan was meaning. 'I'm not sure I know exactly what you mean.'

'Normal, steady, reliable.' He paused. 'Huh,' he spoke the word with some force, 'that's a good one.' He looked Jeannie in the eye. 'Not a strong quality in me, but I want to cultivate it.'

'You seem to be attending sessions here pretty reliably, Dan, but I appreciate that your image of yourself is unreliable.'

Jeannie voices what is for her an authentic view of Dan's commitment to the sessions. It is not meant as a deliberate challenge as a technique which is not a person-centred way of working; she is simply being open and honest about her experienced perception of Dan being quite reliable in attending the sessions.

That took Dan by surprise. He was very much of the belief now that he was unreliable. He had been told it enough by his parents in the past, and by Gemma, and, of course, he said it to himself a lot as well. Reliable, he'd got to think of that as predictable and he didn't do predictable, did he? Did he? 'I've thought of myself as unreliable I guess for a while, feels like it's another significant part of me, that. I don't like being predictable, like to do what I like, you know.'

'Mhmmm, don't like to be predictable but rather feel able to do what you want to do.'

'But what I do is, I mean, oh shit. What I do is actually pretty predictable, isn't it?'

'Seems that way to you now?'

'Yeah. It does. I guess addicts are pretty predictable creatures. I thought I wasn't, thought I was making my own choices, doing my own thing, but I wasn't really, just following along, doing what others did. And now I've been getting predictable in other ways, playing those computer games, for instance, not being helpful at home. You think you're being free and making your own choices, but I haven't, just getting into habits, and then changing those habits for different ones.' Dan shook his head. 'Christ, it's depressing.'

'Leaves you feeling depressed, thinking that what you thought was being free was actually about habit, and changing habits.'

'Yeah.' He paused. 'Yeah.' He spoke the word more slowly the second time. 'And habits are so predictable, aren't they?'

'Mhmmm.'

Dan thought about his life, reflecting back over how it had been. A lot he hadn't a clear memory of any more, all a bit drugged up and hazy, but predictability was a feature. 'Thinking about my life, about how predictable some of it has been.'

'Goes back a long way then?' Jeannie was aware that this wasn't really empathising with Dan, but her sense was that he was looking a bit distant as though he had gone a long way back within himself.

Jeannie's response does have reasoning to it and although it is not a simple attempt to direct Dan back to early life, it may well have that effect should he choose to do so. Often it is not so much what is said as the intention or reasoning behind it that indicates whether a therapist's response is related to what the client is communicating or whether it is simply some unconnected comment that is more a reflection of the counsellor's agenda than anything else. Obviously, such comments when they are of the latter type are not an application of the person-centred approach.

'I was thinking back to childhood, you know, and to my father. He was so bloody predictable with his drinking and how he was when he got back. In one sense we didn't know what would happen next, but in a sense we did. Same arguments, same atmosphere. Like a ritual, coming home drunk, arguing with my mother, sometimes something got smashed, sometimes it got violent as well, but it was just a continuous routine, and we would sit there listening to it, not knowing what to do, feeling frightened and . . . , well, just frightened.'

'Mmm, predictable routine and you were left frightened with your brothers.'

'Makes me feel sad and angry thinking about it now.'

'Mhmmm.' Jeannie nodded her head. 'Really sad, really angry.'

'Yeah.' Dan could feel himself tending more towards the anger than the sadness, anger towards his parents, but particularly towards his father. He could feel his chest tightening and his breathing had changed, his fists were clenching. 'Yeah, really fucking angry.' His jaw had tightened now and his arms and shoulders had tightened as well. Jeannie noticed this as well.

'Anger in your heart, anger in your body.'

'There are times when I wish I could have just punched his fucking lights out. But what could we do? Now, I see him as he is, and he's not the person that he was. He's changed a lot. But I still remember how it was and I still feel the anger when I think about it, and what effect it had on me, on us.'

'That effect on you and your brothers, that really gets to you.'

'Yeah.' Dan took a deep breath. 'Yeah, and I feel so ...' Dan couldn't find the words to describe how he felt. He just knew he was bubbling with what felt hot and fiery. It burned inside him. 'Sometimes I just want to explode.' He shook his head. 'But I think I'm afraid to.'

'Afraid to explode?' Jeannie was aware of feeling very concentrated as she listened to Dan, sensing this to be a really important part of the session.

Dan took another deep breath. 'Yeah, my father would lose his temper, sometimes at us. Sometimes he would hit us. Haven't thought about this in the longest while. But it's kind of clear to me again right now. He'd lose it and lash out, usually with the back of his hand. We weren't always quick enough. I remember seeing him hit Tony once, knocked him flying. Fucking bastard. He literally knocked him off his feet, landed under the kitchen table.' Dan shook his head. 'Lucky he didn't hit his head.'

'Terrible to watch.'

Dan nodded. He could see the scene now: his father turned and walked out, slamming the door; his mother in tears trying to comfort Tony; while he and Jake, after getting over the momentary shock, were running to their mother. He remembered them all huddled under the kitchen table; they were all crying. He must have been about eight or nine, Tony was a little younger, Jake a bit older, but they were all crying.

'Yeah.' Dan didn't describe the scene in his head. 'Probably more than any other experience that one set me off.'

'Set you off?'

'Using, sniffing. Just tried to keep out the house as much as I could really. Nothing there for me any more. Always felt so tense at home, couldn't relax, just needed to get away from it, you know, and not just get away from being in the home, being away from the mess in my head, from the ...' He sighed. 'Oh, I don't know, the everything.'

'So being out and sniffing kept you away from the tension and the mess in your head.' Jeannie was aware of feeling suddenly very sad for this little eight-year-old boy having to keep away from a place that should have been full of love and full of safety. She was aware that her lips had tightened.

'Had to get away, had to.' Dan paused. 'Just had to.'

'Just had to get away.' Jeannie spoke softly, not wanting her words to disturb Dan's own focus on his internal experiencing.

Sometimes empathic responses can disrupt the internal flow of experiencing within the client, however accurate and well-meaning they may be. Spoken softly, yet clearly, they can be heard by the client but in such a way that they provide a kind of background reassurance that they have been heard rather than something external to themselves that they feel drawn in the moment to place their primary attention upon.

Dan closed his eyes. It had been a hard time. A very empty time, full of feeling alone although he had his friends. But they didn't take away that feeling inside himself. He could feel himself so small as he connected with these feelings that although 20 years had passed, nevertheless the feelings seemed as real today as they had then. He realised that he was crying, that tears were trickling down his cheeks.

'But I never really could, it was always in my head. Always in my head.' Dan shook his head. 'And then there was Billy, and you know about that.' More tears flowed and Dan slumped back in the chair, raising his right hand to his face and supporting his elbow with his other hand. He had his fingers and thumb across his eyes, his head bent slightly forward. His body convulsed as the tears continued to flow.

'Yeah, I know about that.'

Dan continued to cry for what seemed to Jeannie like an age but she did not waver in her attention. And she did not feel anything other than an overwhelming sense of compassion and of wanting to reach out to him.

'I just felt so empty inside, so empty.'

Jeannie got up and walked over to where Dan was sitting and as she looked down on him, he looked up, their eyes met and she instinctively reached out to hold him. He held her tightly, crying like a baby, heart-wrenching sobs that she felt against her body, his body hot against hers. She held him tightly back, empathising with his physical need to hold and be held. They stayed in that position for some minutes with nothing more being said.

Jeannie's impulse to move over to Dan has emerged out of her compassion for him. Whether she was planning physical contact, or simply offering the opportunity, only she will know. Either way, something spontaneous occurred and has left them in physical contact, Dan distraught and Jeannie holding him. When does a counsellor initiate physical contact with clients, or do they leave the client to seek it? What are the boundaries? For many people, the need to feel held, and without any sexual component, is hugely important and responding to this need can prove to be amazingly therapeutic and beneficial. However, the person-centred counsellor, and indeed any counsellor, needs to do a reality check. Where are they coming from in the moment? Sometimes they will know, but often they will not. The act will be a simple human response from one person to another, the therapist feeling moved to reach out.

The challenge for the person-centred counsellor is whether they can trust the therapeutic process by responding in this way. In a world in which there seems an increasing risk of complaint, it is often the truly courageous counsellor who will be willing to take the risk. This is sad. Clients have to be protected, yes, but so often the simple spontaneous act of a physically reassuring hug can convey more empathy, unconditional positive regard and genuineness than any spoken word.

Finally, Dan began to ease his grip on Jeannie. 'Oh God.' He let her go.

She sat by him on her haunches. 'OK?'

'Yeah.' He blew out a long breath and reached for a tissue. 'Yeah. Thanks.'

'You just seemed to need to be reached out to.'

He nodded. 'Yeah, then and now. Felt like you reached out to both of us.' He closed his eyes and breathed deeply again, blowing it out once more. 'Yeah, I really needed that. Like, yeah, felt good, felt so good.'

Dan was aware of feeling a little spaced out in his head. He blinked. 'Feeling a bit buzzy, bit spaced.' He blinked again.

'Take your time. You were experiencing some powerful and distressing feelings back there.'

'Tell me about it!'

'We have only a few minutes left; how do you want to use them?'

'Just sit quiet for a moment or two first.' Dan reached over to the glass of water on the table and took it; resting back into the chair he began to sip from it. It had been a powerful experience. He had really felt held, really held, probably for the first time in his life. It had been so ... He thought about what would describe it but the words that came to mind didn't capture the experience. It had felt releasing, uplifting, reassuring. It was painful; he had felt like he was being torn in two, like a volcano bursting under the force of the burning, molten lava. He couldn't put it into words though really; it was all of these things and more.

Jeannie was now mindful that the time to end the session had arrived. 'You released a lot there, Dan, and I guess you will need to just take care of yourself for a little while as it may have left you very sensitive.'

Dan acknowledged this, they confirmed the time of the next appointment and he left, still feeling a little spaced but generally feeling reassured at some deep level, and the thought that kept coming to his mind was that he was OK. He really was OK.

After the session, and when she had got home, Jeannie's thoughts turned to a piece she had read some while back, called *The Jigsaw of Self*. She knew she had a copy somewhere and went to look for it. She read it through (see p. 119).

Points for discussion

- How do you interpret Dan's switch from talking about blaming himself to talking about his tiredness and his methadone use?
- Critically assess Jeannie's work in Sessions 11 and 12.
- What feelings and thoughts do you hold for the configurations that emerged during these sessions? Can you feel warm acceptance to them all and, if not, what implications does this have for you as a counsellor?
- Would you have described your thoughts at the start of Session 12? Did it have therapeutic value?
- How do you react to the jigsaw metaphor? What other metaphors might have more meaning for you in describing this process?
- What are the implications of Jeannie holding Dan when he was so distraught towards the end of Session 12?

Summary

Dan talks about his life at home and his struggle to cope with normal everyday things. He talks of his need to do what he wants, how the computer games absorb him. Jeannie struggles with her empathy. Dan talks about feeling small inside a big body. He talks from his 'little boy blue' configuration of being lost in a green fog and 'the addict' configuration emerges, almost with its own identity. Configurations and dissociated states are briefly contrasted. Dan explores himself using the metaphor of a jigsaw. It dawns on him how predictable he is, and how challenging that recognition is for him. He experiences anger, particularly towards his father. He connects with deep feelings of sadness and describes an incident when his father assaulted his younger brother and how that triggered his sniffing. Jeannie holds Dan as he cries and releases pent-up feelings.

The Jigsaw of Self by Richard Bryant-Jefferies

It is my belief that we, as human beings, have greater potential to resolve our own difficulties and problems than we are often credited with. I believe that our life experience can often undermine our sense of self, leaving us weak and unconvinced of our own abilities. I have recently been reflecting on the image of a jigsaw as representing the person, the sense of self that we carry with us into each new day, yet which is constructed on the basis of past experience, much of which damages our sense and experience of self.

I am convinced that we begin our lives with many potentials and talents. These may (or may not) develop and find expression as we move through life's experiences. Their emergence can be hindered as we develop a view of ourselves based largely around the opinions and feedback we receive from significant others, some of which generates a negative self-concept or poor self-image. We may find ourselves conditioned into ways of being, into ways of behaving and of seeing ourselves that are more concerned with fulfilling other people's expectations than discovering our own worth and genuine self-expression. We can think of this as being represented by a jigsaw whose pieces have been put together in such a way that the overall picture cannot be seen, creating a disjointed image that does not measure up to our full worth as a person. We are often caught up in putting much of our energy into creating someone else's picture rather than our own.

If we think of ourselves (albeit rather simplistically) as a jigsaw put together over the course of our lives, many of us will feel, I am sure, that we have got some of the bits in the wrong places. If the jigsaw represents our sense of self then we may continue putting down pieces in places that, while producing an image of colours and shapes, obscures our potential as a fully functioning person. We cannot be the person we have the potential to become if the pieces do not seem to fit together in a way that makes us feel whole and fully present. We may be left with a feeling of inner fragmentation.

Of course, we may go through life accepting our sense of self, the image that we have created metaphorically in the jigsaw, subtly conditioned into believing it to be a truthful representation of who we are or, rather, of who we have become. And in a real sense, it is truthful. We can feel congruent to that image, seeing it as a mirrored reflection of how we see and experience ourselves, and confirmed to us through the feedback that we receive from those around us. Our 'locus of evaluation', as Carl Rogers termed it (1961, p.354), has become centred outside ourselves, invested in the opinion of others. We may continue to function well in this condition, feeling comfortable with the sense of self that we have created, even if it is obscuring our ability to engage with a state of fuller functionality as a person.

Yet we also know that many of us enter into a phase, or phases, of life when we question our sense of self; times when we begin to wonder whether we truly are being ourselves or living out the hopes, expectations, dreams and fears of the significant others that make such a deep impression upon us. It may be that the person that we have identified ourselves as being for so long, the self-concept that we have created for ourselves, is somehow not working or coping any more; we may be breaking down under the pressure that life's demands have placed upon us. Or we may feel an overwhelming sense of being constrained by patterns and habits of living that somehow we no longer find as satisfying as they once were. We can feel out of step with ourselves, letting the old habits and patterns live on (keeping to the same image of the jigsaw) yet feeling somehow it is not us, that there is something out of place. We are beginning to feel that the image on the jigsaw of self is not as we wish to see ourselves, or feel we want to be. Another way we might experience this is through the sense that life is taking us in a direction that we do not feel is ours to take.

It is at this point that a person may find him or herself facing a crisis of decision:

- whether to shore up the self-concept that has developed over the years and with which they are now so familiar, even though it no longer feels right, in the hope that it will all be OK and that it is just a 'silly phase'
- whether to face the possibility that through conditioning they have lost touch with the potential as a person that they might grow towards becoming.

This may seem a stark and simplistic choice to be made between two extremes. In reality, I believe, they do not exist at extremes in isolation but rather as extreme ends of a continuum. The reality is often that we may wish to accept certain aspects of who and how we have become while questioning other areas of our natures and habits of living. It is often parts of our nature or behaviour that we feel unsure or uncomfortable about although it can be the situation that we are questioning our whole sense of self. We may choose to seek help, guidance or direction and this may involve a decision to enter into a therapeutic relationship with another person in which to make sense of and grow through the crisis. It is here that I wish to return to the image of the jigsaw.

Client-centred therapy

There are many approaches to counselling and psychotherapy. I wish to focus on client-centred therapy. It is an approach in which the therapist seeks to communicate empathy, congruence and unconditional positive regard towards the client. The client is offered freedom to explore whatever they wish to focus on without the therapist seeking to make interpretations or judgements as to what choices should, or should not, be made. A core attitude within the therapist is a recognition that the person they are with can be trusted to experience growth where the core conditions are present. Yet it has to be more than a recognition. The trustworthiness of the individual and the core conditions have to be communicated genuinely by the therapist and received accurately by the client. It is not the case with this way of working that the therapist seeks to 'sort out' or 'heal' or 'make better', but rather the intention is to offer a genuine, sensitive and open relationship. It is from this accepting experience that the client may then undergo a psychological process moving them towards healing or resolution of difficulties.

Imagine yourself as the client. You have come along because of difficulties in your life. You are not coping well and you want to make sense of what is going on and to find a solution. In terms of the jigsaw metaphor, the pieces have not been put together as they might have been, and in a way that might have enabled you to feel more whole and genuinely yourself as a fulfilled person.

The therapeutic process begins and you talk about yourself; how you see yourself; the situations you feel you handle well, and those you do not; the highs and lows in your life; your hopes and fears. By talking and exploring these facets of your life and experience you 'externalise' them, you externalise a picture of yourself from which you can begin to see the whole picture that you have created more clearly. You are in a position then to question how some of the pieces have been fitted together. This is not analysis at a distance. Feelings and thoughts are engaged with, and are often lived in the therapy session. What seems to be important is that they are 'put out' and the therapeutic relationship is such that they can be explored, understood and reintegrated, yet with perhaps an added, or different, meaning as a result.

In the therapeutic relationship you find your sense of self changing as you feel heard and listened to, valued and accepted as a person in your own right by someone who is endeavouring to be real and fully present in relationship with you. Pieces of the jigsaw are seen more clearly as being in the wrong place, symbolising those elements within your own nature and self-concept that are the effect of conditioning in your life and which have had a bearing on your self-concept. The safety and trustworthiness of the relationship enables you to explore more freely, experimenting with new ways of being that seem to be more you, releasing emotional and intellectual blocks to change.

The role of the client-centred therapist is not to point out or to suggest which bits to move in the metaphorical jigsaw. This is crucial. The process is concerned with enabling you to trust your own judgement and insight, to believe in the validity of your perceptions and interpretations. You, the client, are trusted to see for yourself. The time to question the placing of a piece within the metaphorical jigsaw of self is when you, the client, acknowledges that it is not right. The therapist will help the exploration of what a piece may mean to you, why it has been placed where it has, why it is no longer seen to fit in with your changing sense of self. The therapist will not, however, tell the client to change it. The piece can only be changed when the client within him or herself knows that it is no longer right, that the facet of themselves that it represents is no longer a sustainable part of their self-image, and that they have begun to develop a sense of what it is to be replaced with.

Limitation and expansion

I do not want to encourage, however, a view that is too rigid of the process of solving or resolving – I am not sure which is the most appropriate word – the jigsaw of self. I am not even sure if it is a linear piece-by-piece process; maybe we get breakthroughs and pieces come together in groups, clumping together to generate a new self-image in a particular area of our life. Perhaps there are sudden shifts as we see ourselves in a fresh light and reinterpret our own experiences from the past and the present. Perhaps these significant changes might be seen to correspond with Carl Rogers' idea of 'moments of movement'. It may even be that in some mysterious way parts of our nature are assembled before they are positioned within our natural way of being, represented by how, when working on a jigsaw, we might group pieces to complete a small section of the picture before introducing it into the larger picture itself. Can this process occur psychologically? Perhaps it can where we act 'as if' we had a particular quality, testing out an element of our potential prior to that final acceptance of 'yes, that really is me'.

Of course, the jigsaw image has its limitations. It may be that it should be thought about in other ways to become a more realistic reflection of the self. I am unsure, for instance, whether the pieces should have fixed shapes, patterns or colours, or whether they may themselves evolve. I also want to know whether there is a limit to the possible number of pieces available, whether we ourselves have infinite possibilities or whether there is a fixed limit to who we can become. I wonder, too, whether the pieces that are considered to be in the wrong places need to be placed elsewhere, or whether they need to be discarded, no longer part of the overall picture. And what does it mean, psychologically, to discard a piece of the jigsaw of self?

I also find myself wondering whether the image itself contains the seeds of new images that will emerge in time, a kind of fractal reality which, when the image is completed, enables the individual to move deeper into themselves or maybe gain a more expansive sense of self. What does 'expansive' mean in this context? Does it indicate greater congruence in the person as they are, or added to this a sense of the potential to become more than their current congruent self?

Could it be that from an early age we contain within us the seeds of our becoming, yet the journey we take and the self we create as we move through life ensures that the final outcome cannot be known until it is reached? Who knows? Is it that in life there is not so much a goal, but more of a direction? Carl Rogers wrote of an 'actualising tendency', an urge to grow towards fuller functionality as a person. Perhaps our experience of the journey through life is more significant than being overly concerned about reaching the goal? I can only wonder as to the undiscovered potentialities of what it is to be a human being.

Towards completion

It may well be a slow process to rebuild the jigsaw of self, or it may prove to be quite rapid. Some people may only need to change a few pieces; others may require a great deal of change, many pieces needing to be moved or removed. It is my belief that by engaging in a client-centred therapeutic relationship the jigsaw of self can change and evolve into a clearer and less distorted image of the person. It may not be possible to get all the pieces in the 'right' places through one series of therapy sessions. Breaks may be needed to assimilate and consolidate the new arrangement, to put it to the test, if you like. It may be that particular areas of the picture are concentrated on as these are areas in which the client is aware of a need to change, or at least to revisit and engage with. It is likely that even by the end of life the jigsaw may not be fully completed. Indeed, we might consider ourselves extremely fortunate if it is! Yet it is my belief that the more we can solve the jigsaw of self, ensuring that more and more of the pieces are appropriately positioned in relation to each other, the greater will be our capacity to live enriching and nourishing lives, and be more of the person that we have the potential to become.

CHAPTER 9

Supervision 3

'So, you have found yourself working with configuration of self with Dan?'

'Yes, and it has been very interesting and I have been surprised by the strength of identity that they have, and it left me wondering what that was about.'

'How do you mean?'

'Well, it was in that session where he really seemed to be talking from two of the configurations, "the addict" and what came to become known as "little boy blue". I was left wondering after the session whether the chemical impact of drug use might somehow affect the potency and individuality of configuration.'

'Interesting thought, and probably not an area that there has been much investigation into.'

'It seemed that the parts of Dan that emerged had something about them that made them seem more like dissociated parts, and yet they weren't, as far as I know, developed out of traumatic experience such as sexual abuse, at least, I assume not. Of course, that could still be a factor that Dan is quite unaware of or not voicing, but I don't think so. But I could be wrong.'

'So maybe it would be helpful to contrast configurations within the Self and dissociated process. Let's see what's written.'

Max reached over to the bookshelf and took down a copy of *Person-Centred Therapy Today* (Mearns and Thorne, 2000). 'Mearns writes of configurations which are established around introjects, dissonant self-dissonant self-experiences and he highlights the presence of what he terms "growth and not-for-growth" configurations (pp.108–116). And, yes, here we are, the chapter by Margaret Warner. She writes that "dissociated experiences ... are a great deal more personified than ordinary mood states or even "configurations" (p.162). And here, "dissociated process seems to arise almost exclusively as a response to early childhood trauma" (p.158). She goes on to say that these dissociated parts "seem to emerge when trauma memories are pressing to the surface" (p.163).'

'OK, but what differentiates them?'

'OK, so what about contrasting the two concepts. Yes, here we are.' Max continued reading. 'Mearns suggests that one key difference is linked to the

" 'protective' function" of the parts, leading, in dissociated process to "some of the 'parts' becoming dissociated from each other to the extent that there is a loss of awareness between parts" (p.108). He also adds that "it is important to note that while the notion of 'configurations' within the Self may bear some similarities with dissociated process, it is not on a continuum with dissociative identity disorder (DID), formerly known as multiple personality disorder. In considering Self in regard to 'configurations', we are embracing 'normal' dimensions of personality integration" (p.108).'

'OK, so no continuum, we are talking about different developments within the Self.'

'Right. He then goes on to refer to Ross (1999) writing about "pluralism within the self not being on a 'dissociative continuum' with DID", and then suggests that there is a "qualitative difference in the *personification* of the parts – the parts may even have 'people' names rather than descriptive titles which is more common in configurations" and that "there is a much more profound *separateness* between the parts" (p.108). So, the personification and separateness of the parts seem to be important factors.'

'And my understanding is that with dissociative process, "parts" can even be unaware of each other.' Jeannie felt she was getting some clarity now on an area that had often been a bit of a mystery.

'Yes, so it seems a matter of degree but with a very definite need to bear in mind the origin, and the important factor of the experience of traumatic child abuse.'

'Hmmm. So, dissociated states are likely to emerge out of early childhood traumatic experiencing, in particular sexual abuse, whereas configurations are a normal development, simply the parts that make up the Self and which we develop and live out of or through as we move through different experiences in life.' Jeannie thought back to her sessions. 'I'm not sure what we have here. I mean, they seemed like configurations, although there has been trauma involved, as I mentioned earlier, yet there does seem to be a distinctiveness. The violence at home may not have triggered a dissociative process but then there may be factors and experiences that Dan has not talked about.'

'Mhmmm.'

'Plus, of course, there is the factor of the chemical use from an early age and what impact that might have had on brain chemistry, neural pathway development and Dan's own direct experience of himself, and therefore on his own processing of parts of himself that had emerged or were to emerge later. Could configurations get more fixed through the kinds of chemicals Dan was using? I don't know. I do just wonder.'

'Something to look up and check out.' He paused. 'Perhaps what is important here is the work you are doing in allowing Dan to appreciate the different parts of himself, whatever their origin, and to provide a safe environment for this to occur.'

'I think safety is a big issue. There is a lot of vulnerability and sensitivity. Dan is showing aspects of himself to me, and in a sense realising them about himself as well. I don't want to get too tangled up in complexity and lose my simplicity of being a companion to his journey into himself.'

Max nodded.

'Whatever the origin of the parts that are present for Dan, he needs a place to bring them – should I say be them – in which all feel equally accepted, yes?'

'Yes.'

'And he must be sufficiently trusting of me and our relationship for him to reveal them, or for them to reveal themselves.'

'Mhmmm.'

'And we know that more parts may emerge, I mean, the number of configurations that could have been developed in response to introjects could be large. And if there is dissociative process at work, there may be parts that have yet to appear of which Dan, and the other parts, are quite unaware.'

'So Dan really needs you to be warmly accepting of him, all of him, to be authentically present and empathically accurate, to offer an opportunity for him to be fully present, or should I say all of him to become fully present.'

'Yes. And I really need to trust his process, don't I? I mean, I know that, but I *really* have to be there.'

'Well, yes, you are going to be operating in the dark, unsure of what might emerge at any time, having to be sensitive and responsive to whatever Dan reveals of himself.'

Such openness is extremely important as Jeannie is seeking to encourage Dan's process of being to become freer and more transparent to her. If the counsellor cannot be open and is not experienced as such by the client, then what they reveal of themselves can be blocked.

'OK. And let me just mention that we also moved towards using the metaphor of a jigsaw, with Dan turning over the pieces and having to decide how to fit them together and which pieces he wanted as components of the person he is striving to become. And we reached the point where he could recognise that he may not know which parts to keep as he has no idea of the final picture.'

'So, pieces represent parts of Dan, and he is basically recognising the pieces and then deciding which to keep and how to fit them together.'

'Yes.'

'I think I need to think about that.' Max paused. 'But you say it seems to be helping Dan make sense of himself?'

'Yes, so I am quite happy to go with that and allow him to process it.'

'Sounds intriguing. The thought strikes me, though, that there is no finished picture, that the metaphor requires that the picture is continually evolving. Dan, or any of us, never reaches a point of full functionality, or do we? Surely he will find that the picture changes as he absorbs new experiences, extracts meaning from them and his sense of self adjusts to his experiencing and the symbolisation process.'

'Hadn't thought of that. But he has realised that his choices and decisions now govern what or how he finally emerges from his process and I think that recognition has had a profound impact on him.'

'That he is responsible for his own process and outcome?'

'Yes, particularly as responsibility hasn't been a quality hugely in evidence, at least, that's what he has indicated.'

'You really are connecting with Dan and working across so much of his sense of self.'

'He has given me a lot since I last saw you, and some very painful and difficult experiences too. Seeing his best friend die in front of him, what a traumatic experience that must have been. I can see that he has a long journey within therapy ahead of him and I think that the work I am doing with him may go the distance, but I may be a companion on part of his journey only.'

'I'm curious why you say that.'

Jeannie thought about it. 'I think it may be a sense of just how much work there may be to do, and maybe I'm avoiding thinking that I am taking it all on.'

'A sense of your own avoidance of so much.'

'Overwhelming. And if I feel overwhelmed at the thought, what must Dan feel? He is faced with so much change and adaptation to really move on and ensure he can achieve what he wants – a sustainable drug-free life. I really do admire him. He seems to be persevering so far. He's a regular attendee, only missed that session when he had lapsed.'

'Yes, he is showing real commitment, and you feel a sense of admiration for him.'

'I do. He's struggling to free himself from patterns and habits.' Jeannie remembered that she had something else she wanted to check out, although it seemed that it may be linked to what they had been discussing. 'There is something else that I want to raise. When I was waiting for Dan at the start of the last session, I got somewhat lost in my own thinking and as a result went out late to find him. I just started reflecting on things related to Dan and before I knew it I was ten minutes into the session. I rather feel now that it is linked to the notion of it feeling overwhelming, so many facets to think about.'

'So you found yourself immersed in thinking about Dan and it feels linked to feeling overwhelmed.'

'The sense that there is so much, so many lines of thought.'

'And the thoughts got in the way of Dan actually coming into the room.' Max knew he was being a little provocative, but he wanted to explore this further.

Jeannie nodded. 'Yes. Yes, stopped him coming in the room, it did, didn't it? Was I protecting myself in some way, I wonder? Last time we talked about me feeling overloaded and what effect that could be having. I guess it is still happening, but has come out in a different way. I'm not aware of having lost focus in the sessions, though. And I'm not feeling tired either talking about him, so something has shifted there as well. But I have to keep my discipline on this.'

'I think it is easy to get caught up in the complexities of theory here, and in a sense we kind of paralleled that earlier. I mean, I don't often get a book off the shelf and start quoting it at supervisees! So, something stirred me up as well, left me feeling a need to do that. Just seems to be something around the complexity of Dan and maybe we are both struggling in different ways to feel, I don't know, on top of it? Does that sound right?'

Jeannie wasn't sure. 'For me it is about feeling able to be open and fully present.'

'Of course, so why do I go and say "on top of it"?'

'Want to explore it? May have some relevance here.' Jeannie was aware of a kind of role reversal but she felt OK with that. It had sounded odd what Max had said and maybe it did have some connection to Dan's complexity.

Roles are reversed and Jeannie has encouraged Max to explore his experience and reaction. After all, they are forming a therapeutic relationship, albeit supervisory in nature, and when the supervisor experiences something relevant it can be usefully explored then and there in the session. In the final analysis, supervisor and supervisee are co-professionals, working together collaboratively.

Max nodded. 'I suppose it is about getting a handle on what is going on, and somehow as I say that I immediately hear a little voice inside myself saying, "so you're not trusting the process". And maybe that's it, I am not trusting the process and for me that is about the chemical impact of the drugs. I know that the actualising tendency will continue to operate, but I just have a sense that there is a chemical barrier and it's making it difficult for me to get a grip on the situation. It feels foggy.'

Jeannie broke out in goosebumps. 'When I saw you last, had I mentioned the green fog?'

'I don't recall that.'

'No, of course, it was the session before last. Dan talked about being in a green fog, holding him back, making him feel stuck, yet keeping him from knowing what was outside of it. Well, he mentioned that "the addict" made him drink it, and it became clear that it had to be the methadone.'

'I'm getting affected by the fogginess? Struggling to get a grip, to, as I said, "get on top of it".'

'Makes sense?'

'Could be that I'm picking up the fogginess. Interesting that you are not tired this session, so you are maintaining clarity, but it is me that is in the fog.' Max was intrigued by all of this. He found the process of supervision fascinating and these kind of experiences always left him with a sense of wonder. He wanted to explore it more, but he knew this was Jeannie's time, and it did seem that they had made sense of it. So he decided he should take it to his supervisor and allow Jeannie the time to continue with what she wanted to bring to their supervision session.

Jeannie appreciated this and went on to talk about the hug she had given Dan and how powerful it had felt. They both acknowledged not knowing what meaning Dan ascribed to it, but that it had had a profound effect. They explored briefly the importance of physical contact being therapeutically justifiable and how difficult that could be when it proceeded out of a sense of therapeutic connectedness with the client, and the risks associated with a client misinterpreting what was intended through the physical contact.

CHAPTER 10

A month later

Dan had attended three sessions, and one he had been away for. They had spent more time focusing on the parts of Dan that seemed to make up his personality, and it had been painful and emotional at times as he released more bottled-up feelings from his past, in particular those linked to Billy's death, his father, and the abuse he and his brothers experienced, and he had also spoken a little more about Jake's death as well.

In himself Dan was aware of feeling a great deal more, but it was still all very uncomfortable; in fact it had seemed to have eased, but the last week had not been easy at all. He was feeling concerned, wondering quite what was happening, and was glad to have the counselling session today. He hadn't used anything other than his methadone script, and was really pleased with that. He was doing things around the house. He was attending AA. He was doing more things with Gemma and her son as a family. But he knew he didn't feel right, and it seemed as though it was getting worse, not better. He really wanted to try and make sense of it all.

Session 16

Dan was on time and he walked quite purposefully towards the counselling room, sat himself down and immediately started talking.

'It's been a difficult week. I think what we have been talking about is stirring me up, and I'm not feeling so confident. I'm continuing with the AA, and that feels good, and I haven't dropped the methadone any further, seem to be stuck at 10 mls. I've talked to Marie, my keyworker, and we may hold off dropping the methadone further just at the moment. I'm not sure what to do, I don't want to stop talking to you, I know it is helpful, but I also want to keep myself kind of stable as well.'

Dan paused and clearly he seemed to have a 'do you have the answer' expression on his face, at least that was how Jeannie saw it. She responded to what he had said.

'Yeah, difficult one, you don't want to stop the counselling but you are concerned that it is leaving you feeling – and the word in my head which you did not use is – vulnerable. Correct me if I'm wrong.'

Jeannie has responded to Dan but used a word that has been very present for her. It is a congruent voicing of her own experiencing arising from her connection with Dan. However, she has voiced it in a way to leave Dan the freedom to correct her.

'No, that sums me up at the moment. I've found myself thinking more about using this week, well, not about using so much as thinking back to when I did use.'

'Mhmmm.' Jeannie didn't say anything more, allowing Dan to continue.

'Some of the feelings I used to get, just feeling, well, no, just not feeling, that's the truth of it. I guess I crave some of the "not feeling" that I used to experience.'

'The not feeling that came from using, yeah?'

Dan nodded. 'Yeah, yeah. And I know it's crazy . . .'

'Crazy?'

'Well, I shouldn't be thinking this way, but I am.'

'So you have certain feelings towards not feeling, and it leaves you thinking that you shouldn't be this way.'

'It just seems that there is a big part . . . well, I don't know, is it a big part? But it feels big at times, a part of me that simply does not want to feel, and the more we have got into feelings, maybe the more that part of me has, I don't know, I guess I'm just more aware of it.'

Jeannie nodded. 'More aware of a "not-feeling" part of you, and it's leaving you feeling . . .?'

'Very vulnerable. Just feel on edge more, like withdrawal but that's crazy, I haven't changed anything just recently, haven't dropped the methadone and have been clear of the alcohol for a few weeks now.'

'So not withdrawing from chemicals or substances . . .' Jeannie let the sentence hang in the air; this was what Dan had said but she was curious as to whether he might feel he is withdrawing from anything else.

'Just feel so on edge, so uptight somehow. Can't seem to settle. I'm actually doing the things we've talked about but I don't feel good. I thought they'd make me feel better.'

'So the changes you made haven't left you feeling good, and that's really troubling you.'

'I expected to feel different, feel more in control, more relaxed, more at ease with myself. I mean, I'm doing what I want to do, I'm being more normal, but I feel sort of . . .' Dan paused as he realised what he was about to say. He grinned.

'You feel sort of . . .?'

'OK, OK, I feel sort of not myself.' He nodded to himself as he said it.

'Not yourself?'

'No, not myself, not the me that I have been. I'm not myself, am I, that's what I'm trying to change.' He shook his head. 'It's like the "not-feeling" me is wanting to take control, yeah, take control.' As he said it Dan could sense a certain irritation with that part of himself. He tightened his lips. 'Yeah.'

'So your experience is that the "not-feeling" part of you is seeking to take control and that is connected to your sense of not feeling yourself.'

Dan has moved to a greater understanding of this 'not-feeling' part of himself, facilitated by Jeannie, who has sought to stay with him using her empathy to communicate what she is hearing him say. By feeling heard Dan has moved in his exploration and his understanding of this 'not-feeling' part.

'I'm not feeling myself because I am trying to not be how I was. I have to accept that I am doing different things but they are provoking reactions, feelings some part of me doesn't like, and sometimes they are good feelings but they get lost in this sense of not being myself.'

'So good feelings are getting lost . . .'

'Yeah, they are, and I don't want that. I want to feel good about myself, about what I do, and I was feeling that way last week, but this week, it feels different.'

'Different.'

'And I don't like it, I don't want it. I want to feel good about what I am doing, but some evenings I struggle with it.' Dan thought back over his week. 'Take Monday. Busy but monotonous day at work. Got home, we ate, and I had said I would sort out a kitchen cabinet door that has been sticking. I did it, although it turned out to be a bit more involved than I had anticipated, but I got it sorted. Now, I should have felt good about it, but I didn't. It was like having done it I closed the door and, well, nothing had changed. Everything looked the same. I didn't have any interest in what I had done.'

'So getting the door sorted just gave you no sense of, what, satisfaction?'

'Just felt "what the heck" about it and . . .' Dan stopped again and then started. 'You know, it really is like a part of me does not want me to feel good, and that sounds awful hearing myself say it, but that is how it feels. Part of me does not want me to feel good.'

Jeannie nodded. 'Yeah, awful to feel that part of you does not want you to feel good.'

'And seems to be stopping me feel good.'

'Not just wanting but actually stopping you feel good.'

Dan nodded. 'And as I say that the thought also comes to mind that it isn't just about stopping me feeling good, there's also something about not wanting to feel? And that comes back to what I was saying earlier and the effect of talking to you.'

'Mhmmm, talking to me triggering off something in you that wants to stop you feeling, the "not-feeling" part.'

Dan thought about what Jeannie had said and it didn't quite feel right. 'You know, not so much "not-feeling" as a "not-for-feeling" part. That somehow makes more sense to me, but I still don't like it, well, not as I sit here now anyway.'

> Dan has been able to clarify his experience of this part of himself further
> through hearing Jeannie's empathic response. It is an important distinction
> that Dan makes, though only Dan will appreciate what this difference is.

'Mhmmm.'
'And I do want to feel, but I don't like some of what I feel. Part of me just wants to
  block everything and get me back to not feeling, being drugged up, out of it.'
Jeannie was aware of her mind lingering on this notion of a 'not-for-feeling' part;
  another configuration, she thought to herself? Certainly sounds like it, and one
  that must have had a dominant part in fuelling the drug use.
'Yeah, block it all out and feel nothing.'

> Jeannie does not voice her thoughts; rather she maintains her empathy with
> Dan. Her thoughts are ahead of where Dan is in himself. She does not want
> her ideas to impact on his own process of thinking through what is happen-
> ing for him.

'I don't want that, Jeannie, I really don't.' Dan paused. 'And yet I do.' His facial
  expression seemed to reflect a certain sense of resigned helplessness. He sighed.
'Really hard to sit with knowing that part of you still does want to drug up and be
  out of it.'
Dan nodded. 'But it isn't that I'm thinking specifically of using, more about
  the effect. Yeah, more about the effect. I know people talk of the importance
  of the ritual element, of preparing the gear, you know, just the whole scene.
  Yeah, I've been there, and I was there for a while after stopping and using the
  methadone. But that's not what it's about in my head. It's the effect, that wonderful sense of "don't give a damn".'

> It is well recognised that there is a strong ritualistic element in drug use, in
> the methodology for obtaining the drugs, preparing the paraphernalia, and
> just the everything about it. It can be incredibly habit-forming, for it is such
> an intense experience preparing for jacking up. It's like the one time when
> drug users really savour anticipation, when it all slows down. Otherwise the
> quick-fix mindset is controlling – impatient, intolerant and hell-bent on get-
> ting that next fix.

'Just allowing yourself to not give a damn.'
'So intense, such a beautiful sensation, oh yeah, such a beautiful way to be.' As he
  spoke Dan could almost experience himself becoming that 'what the heck,
  don't give a damn' state. Yeah, he was back there, in his mind at least, but it

felt more than just a thought, it really did. He could feel the sensations in his body; oh yeah, it was good. Problems? What problems. Everything was just fading, leaving him just feeling so good. He suddenly could hear Jeannie's voice. 'Dan, are you OK, you've been silent now for some while.' He could feel a smile inside himself but it didn't feel like it reached his face, it just stayed within him. Yeah, this was where he was meant to be.

Somewhere deep inside himself Dan could feel a presence, a small voice but not exactly, a kind of nagging feeling that this wasn't right. It began to grow stronger and began to hold his attention, like something was emerging inside himself, coming through the wonderful lethargy that had transported him away. Words formed in his head. 'Dan, get a grip, this is not the way forward, this is the past, the way back.' He felt himself frown; that really had reached his face. He realised he must have closed his eyes at some point; he opened them and saw Jeannie. 'Hi.'

She responded in kind, and added, 'Where have you been?'

'That was weird, I really relived sensations from the drugs. That was powerful. I reconnected with something.' He blinked and shook his head, and moved his shoulders having suddenly realised how stiff he felt. He glanced at the clock. 'How long was I . . .?'

'About fifteen minutes.'

'Did I say anything?'

'No. At first you had your eyes open and you looked like you were just reliving something, some memory, you stayed like that for a while, then you closed your eyes, but most of the time your eyes were open.'

'I don't know what happened but it was like I had used, I really felt like I had smack in my veins. Can that happen?'

'Seems like it. That's what it felt like, yeah?'

'Yeah. I mean I've heard about drinking dreams (Bryant-Jefferies, 2001), you know, waking up feeling you've had a drink, really vivid, when you hadn't, when you were dry. But this was a kind of smack dream, a daydream, but it was for real. Like part of me, the part that holds the memories of what it was like, just took over somehow, some way.'

'Drug-using part?'

'Yeah, and we had been talking about the "not-for-feeling" part, hadn't we, wonder if that was what happened. Could I really be carrying those, well I was going to say feelings, but well, they are more sensations than feelings.' Dan blinked again. 'I really do seem to be opening up to myself, and it feels scary, and it feels necessary as well.' But he looked somewhat bemused by it all.

'You don't look too sure about it.'

'No.' Dan scratched the side of his head. 'No, but it was real and yet it feels dangerous to go there. I mean, I was sitting here, wasn't I, kind of reminiscing and then I just slipped into it.'

'Can you remember it now?'

'Yes, yes I can. But it feels like I'm looking on at it, like the experience was mine but it's kind of, I don't know how to put it, kind of next to me. Like it isn't really inside me, and yet I know it is my experience.'

'So you are in touch with the experience and the sensations, yeah?'

'Yeah. Part of me really doesn't want to let go, does it?'

'That how it seems?'

'Yeah, and I need to let go, I want to let go. It doesn't really do me any good. I still feel hazy, you know, it really has affected me. I really have to break free of the drug use completely, even the methadone. I need to be clean. I want to break free.'

Dan felt emotionally drained, not just emotionally; his whole body suddenly felt heavy as a wave of tiredness swept over him. 'I feel tired, and I want to stay with it, you know?'

'Like experiencing tired just at the moment is important?'

'Yeah. And I feel quite hot too.'

Dan continued to experience his tiredness and struggled with it. In the end he had to say that it was no good, he just felt too whacked and needed to head home. It wasn't the time that the session was due to end, but Dan was struggling to keep awake. Gemma was driving so he went outside to wait, sitting in the cool air which actually helped him to feel a little refreshed, but the tiredness remained. He had felt a little unsteady as he had left the counselling room, it somehow felt airless in the building, but he was determined to find his way through what was happening within him. He was pleased to see Gemma arrive and they headed off. He slept well that night, absolutely flat out.

Jeannie was still feeling some residual anxiety from the period when Dan had sat in silence. She had felt OK about it to begin with but gradually got a stronger and stronger sense of a gulf opening up in the room, as if Dan was somewhere that she couldn't reach. She had been talking to him, calling his name, for some time before he had finally re-emerged from his reliving of his heroin use. She wasn't sure quite what to make of it, but it did seem to her that perhaps his 'not-for-feeling' part had asserted itself in some way. She wasn't sure. She found it confusing at times and she didn't want to analyse it too much, but rather accept that Dan's process was taking him where he needed to be and that she needed to convey her warm acceptance. It's like, she thought, this part just doesn't want him to grow or change, wants to hold him back. I guess it's probably scared, feeling under threat. But then she recognised that even with change, configurations could adjust and adapt, surviving in fresh guises.

Session 17

Dan phoned about ten minutes before the start of the session. The car wouldn't start. Seemed that the battery had died, no power, and he couldn't do anything about it until the next morning, though he planned to try charging it up over night. He apologised to the receptionist and asked if he could speak to Jeannie on the phone. Jeannie came out to the phone. Dan explained the situation and said that he wanted to apologise and say a couple of things, but then he would have to go and get the battery out and charge while it was still daylight.

'It took me a whole day to get over that last session; I was still feeling lethargic the
next day and into the day after. The more I think about it, the more I am sure
that the part of me that wants to hold me back was getting to me. Yes, I know
that part of me is apprehensive about change, of how well I will cope once I am
completely drug-free, but I have to get there and find out.'
'Dan, I really do hear your motivation and apprehension, yeah, must feel pulled
in two directions.'
'More like I'm pulling in one direction with a heavy weight trying to stop me.'

Jeannie completely misses how Dan is experiencing it, but he corrects her.
She has projected how she thinks she might feel and it is not Dan's experience. It is important to stay with what the client is saying, although, as in
this case, clients will help you to appreciate their inner world when they
really want you to.

Dan had really felt what he was describing, yeah, dragging that bloody weight
around. At times it felt really depressing. Would he ever really feel free of his
past, and of the parts of himself that seemed to want to just keep it alive, and
him half dead as a result? It could leave him quite low sometimes. He hadn't
mentioned this to Jeannie, but as he stood there holding the phone, conscious
that he needed to get on and charge that damned battery, he realised that he
did need to say something, but not now. He had to get on. 'Look, I really must
get the battery sorted, Jeannie, in case it does just need charging, though I
think I'll be replacing it tomorrow.'
'OK, no problem. I appreciate your calling me to let me know. OK for same time
next week?'
'Yes. That's fine. See you then, and sorry again.'
'That's OK, and I hope you get the battery sorted OK.'
'So do I. Bye.'
'Bye Dan.'
Flat battery, Jeannie thought, wasn't it Carl Jung who had written about
synchronicity? She wondered whether lack of energy in the battery was a
reflection in some strange way of Dan's lack of energy in that last session, and
maybe some weird manifestation of the part of himself that was holding him
back, the heavy weight he had talked about. She smiled to herself, not convinced about it, and yet ... strange coincidences did happen in life, or were
they only coincidences in the mind of the beholder projecting meaning onto
them, and then taking meaning back out of them? She went to jot down in her
notes that she and Dan had had a brief conversation and then she prepared to
head off home.

Points for discussion

- How would you differentiate a 'not-feeling' part from a 'not-for-feeling' part? Speculate on the different associated behaviours and experiences that might be associated with each.
- What significant moments occurred in the session, allowing Dan to connect with fresh understanding, and how were they facilitated?
- If clients experience vivid dreams or daydreams as happened to Dan, what risks do they carry for the client?
- What was the tiredness about?
- How would you have felt working with Dan when he lapsed into silence and then closed his eyes? How long would you leave him looking like he might have gone to sleep?

Summary

Dan engages with the idea of having a 'not-feeling' part of himself which he redefines as a 'not-for-feeling' part. Jeannie seeks to maintain close empathy with him, allowing him to explore and deepen his understanding. It leads him into a silence in which he relives sensations from his heroin-using days, vivid sensations that he speculates as being like a drinking dream, only a smack dream. He ends the session feeling very tired and leaves early. The next session he does not attend; the car battery is flat. Jeannie reflects to herself on the synchronicity of this.

CHAPTER 11

The past relived; attempting to stop the methadone

Session 18

Dan began by talking about work. He had been asked to take on more work, bit of overtime, and he knew that he could do with the money, but he was unsure. He was still struggling and couldn't make his mind up, but he had to decide by tomorrow. They spent the first part of the session exploring this and Dan still couldn't decide. He wanted to make the decision based on the person he was seeking to become, not the person that he was. He knew that his old self would have had the attitude of 'fuck it, don't do any more than you have to', but he didn't want to be that way, but he also wasn't sure if he felt OK enough to take it on.

'It could mean missing some AA meetings and I may have to make choices between AA and seeing you, and I would prefer to come here.'

Jeannie had allowed Dan to explore this choice further and as a result he had finally decided that he would take on some of the extra work, but not all of it. That, it seemed to him, was a reasonable compromise. He could work late a couple of evenings in the week and Saturday mornings, still get to a couple of AA meetings and get to his counselling. He had talked it through with Gemma, who was of the opinion that he needed to do whatever would help him get better. In fact, Gemma was struggling with Dan's mood and was actually a bit relieved that he would be out a little more in the evenings, but she hadn't said that for fear of making his mood even lower.

'OK, that feels like I have a decision, and I guess I can only see how it goes, you know?'

'Yeah, take it a day at a time, or week at a time, and see how you feel.'

Dan nodded. He blew out a deep breath. 'But it is hard. I still don't feel how I want to feel; my mood, I haven't really talked much about it to you, but it does feel low. I talked to the doctor and he mentioned going onto anti-depressants. I don't want to, but I'm becoming increasingly concerned that I may have to. Just seem stuck. Can't shift into a higher gear. Feel like I'm stuck in first most of the time, occasionally getting into second.'

Lowering mood can be a feature of changing addictive habits, partly because there is a loss involved, and partly the adjustment to the lack of a substance in the system. Often, mood will dip and then begin to pick up after a few weeks. Dan, however, has been struggling for some while and seems to be indicating that it is getting worse. This could be indicative of an underlying depression that has been masked by drug use and which breaks through, or comes to be recognised for what it is, after significant changes in the drug use.

Anti-depressants can help clients gain that lift in mood to help them feel motivated to make changes to their lifestyle and routines. These, once established, then contribute to a raised mood and so the medication can then be reduced. But they can also interfere with the therapeutic process, affecting the degree to which aspects of Dan can be present and be communicated.

The person-centred counsellor will work with as much of the person as can be available, recognising that medication can limit this, but nevertheless offering the core conditions to the person that is present.

'Stuck in first, occasionally in second.'

'I don't know, I don't want to take anti-depressants. I want to be free of it all. I don't want to have to rely on something else. I'm pissed off that I'm still having to rely on the methadone.' He breathed out heavily. 'And I want to be realistic. I'm going to talk to Marie about it when she gets back from annual leave, I don't see her next week, and then decide what to do.'

'You don't want those anti-depressants, don't like having to rely on something . . .' She didn't get a chance to finish.

'No, that's me in the past. I don't want that. I hate it, and yet I'm having to accept it. Shit.' He shook his head. 'I really do want to move on, Jeannie. How many times have I said that here, and I still feel stuck.'

'Feels like you just keep saying it but nothing changes?'

'No, well, I mean, no, things have changed but not enough. Not e-fucking-nough!' Dan brought his fist down on to the arm of the chair. He could feel the utter frustration suddenly build inside himself.

'Not e-fucking-nough change!' Jeannie matched Dan's intensity in her own voice.

Dan's jaw had tightened. 'No.' His teeth were clenched. 'No, and I cannot go on like this.' A memory came to him. 'You remember that green fog I talked about, oh, some sessions back.'

'Yes, how it thickened in the mornings and thinned during the day, and you couldn't see your way forward in it.' Jeannie conveyed what she remembered, wanting to affirm to Dan that she had listened and heard.

'Well, I'm fucking well still in it. Sorry about my language, but it gets to me.'

'That's OK, say it as it is, it fucking gets to you.'

'Yeah. I want to get my head clear, you know, and I know I need the methadone, but I'd really like to get off it and get clean. I think I'm kind of needing to do this more and more, and since going to AA. I mean, I'm clear of the alcohol and feel good about that. I think I've done really well. I know I've done well. But I may be sober but I'm not clean, not while I'm still on that script. I've come down now from 35 mls, gradually reducing and, yeah, I know I had that problem when I dropped the bottle, and shit that was scary. But I want to get clean. And I can feel this need within me and yet I know I have to keep taking it. It's really frustrating, though I also know it is helping me to function as I am sure without it I'd react badly.'

Jeannie sought to empathise with the feelings Dan had conveyed. 'It's really frustrating for you, wanting to get clean but knowing you have to take it to function.'

'Yeah, I mean, it's not like my drugs in the past, you know?' Dan shook his head. 'I've had some bad times, really bad times, particularly when I haven't been able to get any smack. The shakes, aching all over, the shits, sweats, awful, and I don't want that again. But I want to get off and get clean. Guess I need to keep taking it slowly, right. I'd really like to get off it soon, though.' Dan was aware that it was Jake's birthday the start of next week, or at least, it would have been. But he wasn't going to be clear by then. Anyway, he thought to himself, that's all in the past now. Move on.

'Bad withdrawals, yeah? I really do appreciate your urgency in wanting to get off and your realisation that you have to take it slowly.'

'Yeah. That's how it has to be.'

Dan seemed to Jeannie to be accepting of this although it felt like a certain degree of resigned acceptance. She nodded in response to what Dan had said. A silence ensued. Dan wasn't sure what he wanted to say now. He introduced what he was doing at AA and how he was finding it helpful, particularly the feeling of being made so welcome and just having people he could relate to who understood him. He expressed his appreciation not only for them, but also for Marie, his keyworker, the prescribing doctor and Jeannie. He said how he felt sure that without all the support he had had he would have slid back into using again.

In a sense Dan is here denying what he has contributed to his process of recovery. Yes, it is highly likely that without all the support he would have gone back to using, but he has used the support, he has attended counselling, keyworking sessions, appointments with the prescribing doctor and AA meetings. The person-centred counsellor may respond by acknowledging what the client feels, and they may also want to express their own perspective, which will convey appreciation to the client of the effort they have shown. Such prizing is therapeutically valuable when authentically experienced and genuinely offered.

The session then moved into a focus on Dan's drug-using days. Mentioning how awful the withdrawals had been had brought some of it back to him again. He talked about some of the people who had died around him as well. 'But I kept on using. Well, part of the risk I suppose, part of the thrill as well, not knowing, you know, not knowing what you were jacking up.' He shook his head. 'We'd start in the morning, usually had enough between us for the first hit, then when it had worn off and we felt able, we'd go out, either buy some more or maybe go thievin'. There was this one shop near us, I think that woman on the till must have been short-sighted or something. We'd come out with all sorts of stuff. And we'd do a few car radios as well. We knew a guy who'd buy them and sell them on. We didn't care. Or if we saw a bag lying around, we'd just take it. Anything was fair game. Well it had to be, we needed the money to buy the gear. It was a full-time occupation.'

'Yeah, not much time for much else.'

'Nah, not during that phase, what mid- to late teens and into my twenties. Got caught a few times and banged up, occupational hazard. Could still get it though inside, well some of the time. Had to go without one time, shit that was bad. Ended up in the prison hospital. I was bad. But got over it and when I came out, first thing, round me mates and started up again. It was what I did. Nothing else quite like it, you know? Couldn't sit there watching them and not do anything myself.'

'So a few times inside, and generally kept using except that time when you ended up in the hospital.' Jeannie was aware she was simply empathising with his memories, not his thoughts or feelings, but that was what Dan was presenting so she accepted it, acknowledging to herself that, for whatever reason, at this time he wanted to talk about this and presumably wanted her to hear about it as well.

'One time, we'd seen this telly outside this shop, in the fucking high street, just sitting there, don't know why. Guess it was being delivered or something. Mick and I, we looked at each other, didn't have to say anything, just calmly picked it up and walked off, kept walking, never looked back, never stopped till we'd turned a corner. Fucking crazy, but it bought us a supply for a few days, you know.' Dan shook his head. 'If it wasn't nailed down it was ours.'

'Sums it up, huh, if it wasn't nailed down . . .'

'Needed it, had to pay for the habit, had to. But never rented, never did that. Some of the girls went on the game, but never bent over that far! No, not my scene. But some did. Alan did, but he died. Never did really know what happened. Fell in the river. Got fished out but he was dead. Don't know if he fell or was pushed. No one saw it, or no one said anything. You know they've gone but, yeah you're sorry, yeah, but it happens and life goes on.'

'So you could feel sorry but it didn't affect you.'

'No. Not at that time. We were living in squats, sometimes we'd be around some-one's house or flat, but there was always the risk of getting busted. Kept on the move a bit, different places, always able to find the dealers though. Never a pro-blem.' Dan was feeling quite proud of it all, knowing how he'd survived it and, yeah, done what he needed to do. But he had regrets too, now that he looked back, now that he was more in touch with his feelings.

'Always get what you wanted, then?'

'Hmmm? Oh, yeah.' He realised he had drifted off into his thoughts.

'Looked like you were lost in your thoughts for a moment there.' Jeannie had picked it up and wanted to respond to the fact that Dan's hesitancy had conveyed this to her.

'Yeah. I kind of feel good about it in one way, but not good in another.'

'Wish it hadn't happened?' As Jeannie said it she wondered where it had come from. That wasn't a response to anything Dan had said; she wondered if it was her agenda, decided to ponder on it after the session.

'Can't imagine it not happening, you know? Such a big part of my life, part of me. Can't imagine it not having happened.'

'Mhmmm, hard to imagine.'

Dan nodded. He just could not imagine how his life might have been. He couldn't remember a time when he wasn't using. All so much part of his life. Dan just sat and wondered just how it might have been. What would it have been like? He thought back.

'I guess I have to go back to what would have happened if I hadn't started, you know, right at the start – smoking, sniffing, drinking. It was the smoking first. Made me feel different.'

Jeannie knew the importance of that early experience of a drug, any kind of drug.

Many young people regard alcohol, tobacco and illicit drugs as constituting one world of experience rather than separate domains (Advisory Council on the Misuse of Drugs, 1998). It is generally the legal drugs that provide the gateway into the world of illicit drug use. It has been suggested that the under-age consumption of alcohol is a precursor to smoking and the use of other illicit drugs (Society for the Study of Addiction, 1999); however, we should not disregard the role of solvents, which provide a short and intense mood-altering reaction.

'Different, that was important?'

'Oh yeah. Felt, well, felt grown up but also felt buzzy in the head, lot more subtle than what came later, but that was where I first got that sensation. Yeah, haven't thought about that for a long time, but it was where it started. I felt different and it was a good feeling. I know I coughed and choked when I first started inhaling, but I was determined. My mates smoked and I kind of guess that being brought up in a smoky household – my parents smoked heavily – maybe I was already used to it. My lungs had been getting ready for it I guess since I was born.'

'So, cigarette smoking gave you that first buzzy sensation in your head?'

'Yeah, and, well, we got into sniffing I guess because it was happening and it's what you did, you know? Had to have a go, wanted to see what it felt like and, yeah, felt good but it didn't last. Had to keep doing it, walking around sniffing, getting that buzzy, light kind of feeling. It was good. Took my mind off the crap at home. I . . .' Dan was feeling quite connected to his past now. 'I kind of think it was something I felt in control with. I could make myself feel good, and that was important. I felt fucking bad at home, and here was a way I could feel good. And not just me, we all did it, we all had problems I think, not sure about that, maybe some just did it because we were doing it, I don't know. But it was good.'

Jeannie knew she had no experience herself to draw on, she simply had what Dan was telling her. In a way, that made it easier for her to empathise; her own experience wouldn't cloud her clarity of hearing what was being said by Dan.

Does having a background of using the drugs that clients talk about help you to become a better counsellor? Some will argue yes, others no. Perhaps the truth is that you have to decide on an individual basis. It depends what effect a person's drug use has had on them, how much they have dealt with it and how much it remains present for them and easily triggered into memory by what they hear from others. It can help some clients feel that the person they are speaking to understands. To a degree they do, but it will still be their version and the temptation can be that the counsellor who has used in the past will make assumptions as to what the client is seeking to convey, or will not empathise with something because they know what the client means and so don't communicate back their understanding of what the client has sought to convey.

'Felt good, gave you some relief from the crap at home and a sense of having control, of being able to make yourself feel good. Sounds like that last bit was really important.'

'Yeah.' Dan was nodding his head. 'Yeah, that was so important now that I think back to it. So important. Making myself feel good.' As Dan dwelt on that, Billy's face came clearly into his mind. His expression must have changed.

'Mhmmm, and yet it wasn't just good.' Jeannie had noticed Dan's face change from looking quite positive and bright to being suddenly dulled and heavy. She didn't know why, but he had communicated this change and she had wanted to acknowledge it.

'Just thought of Billy.' Dan could feel sadness in himself once more. He took a deep breath through his nose and blew it back out. 'It wasn't good. Think I stopped sniffing because I kept seeing Billy, and the sniffing didn't get rid of it or the feeling, but the alcohol did.'

'Sniffing wasn't powerful enough to stop you seeing Billy, but alcohol, that was something else.'

'Yeah, and we'd sometimes get a joint as well, from Mick's brother. We'd pass it round. Yeah.' Dan shook his head while he smiled. 'That was something else again. Got us into trouble once. Got drunk, but we were actually stoned, and got suspended. Never got excluded though.' Dan shook his head. 'If I had been, well, it would have made things worse. Bad enough when I was suspended.

Spent the week just messing around. Mick was suspended too. Just drank a bit
more, kept out of everyone's way. Now they exclude kids all the time. Yeah, OK,
so they need to show the teachers a bit of respect, but what the hell use is
excluding them? More time on the street. Exclusion – heard someone call it
"state-legitimised truancy". I like that. Just causes more problems for the kids.
Most of them are bored shitless, don't see any point to it all, just want to get a
job and have some fun. Girls just seem to want kids. Boys just want to fuck.
Well, we did, don't suppose that's changed much.'
Jeannie didn't want to encourage a debate on the value or not of exclusion, but
she did want to acknowledge what he had said. 'So, don't see exclusion as helping the kids, and if it had happened to you it would have made things worse,
you reckon?'
'Yeah, just had more time to hang out, yeah. But it didn't come to that. But I never
did much work at school, mucked about, did a little, got by. Didn't care for it or
about it much.'
'School didn't mean a lot to you, just did what you needed to do to get by.'
'Yeah, couldn't wait to leave. Couldn't wait. Wanted to get away from school,
from home, from every-fucking-thing.'
'Mhmmm, just get away, yeah, school, home, everything?'
'Yeah. Then Jake, and my career as a smackhead. Smoked that for a few years,
you know, chasing mostly. Told you this before but it feels important to talk
about it again. I think I feel different now. Think before I was still kind of reminiscing about it; now, well, it's the thought of what my life might have been like
if I hadn't started using. Guess I might have done better at school, but hard to
say. Like at home, you know? Don't think I could have really done well. Too
much chaos in my head without the drugs and the drink. But who knows?
Maybe I'd have got a better job. Maybe I'd have made something of it. But
never really that interested. Always a means to an end, though never enough,
so the thieving had to happen.'
Jeannie nodded. 'Just don't know how things would have turned out, how you
would have become.'
'No, think I'd still be the same person, still messed up, but maybe with a better job
and my own place by now. But then maybe I'd still have drifted into drugs.
More money may have meant more drinking perhaps and maybe still meet
people, you know, ready to sell you what you want. I don't know.' Dan could
feel himself becoming tired, and part of it was feeling tired about the drugs and
about his life. 'Tired of it all, just tired of it all. Want to leave it behind.'
Jeannie empathised with the last things that Dan had said. 'Tired of it all, want to
just put it all behind you.'

It's not necessary or always helpful to seek to convey empathy for everything said by a client. Sometimes the client talks at length and in the journey
arrives at a different place in themselves or perspective on something to
where they had started out. Sometimes the person-centred counsellor will
empathise with the journey, but often may simply respond to the place that

> the client has reached, speaking briefly and allowing the client to continue and to develop whatever it is that they are communicating.

'That's where I am with it. And that's what I'm taking away with me tonight. Thanks, Jeannie, it's been good talking and realising that I am in a different place. I'm not feeling good about the past, not really. I mean, I joke a bit about it, but actually I do feel sad about it all and ... yeah, that's how it ... I feel sad about it all. And I want to change. I really want to change.'

Jeannie reflected this back to Dan, acknowledging the shift he had made in his attitude and that she recognised it too. He said that he appreciated it, that it wasn't just him sensing a shift.

He left, having arranged to attend the following week, but slightly later as he had to go on a training day out of the area, something to do with how to lift things without doing yourself damage.

Jeannie sat back at the end of the session. Dan had gone over his past drug use, well, some of it anyway, and seemed to be different in the way she experienced him talking about it. Thinking back now there did seem to be more regret in his voice. She wondered how it would leave him feeling, but that could only be her speculation. He had felt OK and pleased that he sensed a positive shift in himself. She did ponder on her response about wishing it hadn't happened and now realised that she was probably tuning into something that was present but Dan hadn't really appreciated. But the session seemed to have moved him towards more of a sense of wishing it hadn't all happened. She felt good about that shift.

Session 19

Dan did not look at all well when Jeannie went out to the waiting room to find him.
'Hi Dan, come on through.'
'He got up slowly, and what looked rather painfully, and followed her to the counselling room. 'What's been happening, Dan?'
'Messed up.'
'Messed up.' Jeannie didn't ask him what had happened, thereby offering him the opportunity to stay with how he was feeling.

> It would have been so easy to ask about what had occurred but this would be a directive intervention and not person-centred.

'Yeah, feel like shit.' Dan didn't really feel like saying much. He knew he needed to come to this session, and Gemma had really pushed him, but he knew he just wanted to be in bed and forget everything.

'That bad, huh?'

Dan nodded. He sat feeling so wretched. He hadn't expected this. Last week he had felt so positive, so much clearer, and now ... He sighed to himself. 'Yeah, messed up real good and, I dunno, what's the point. I'm a fucking addict and I'll always be one, won't I? Just can't keep away from using something.'

Jeannie was very aware of not knowing what had happened, but she continued to quell any curiosity and stayed with Dan. 'That's how it feels, you're an addict and you just have to use something?'

Dan didn't reply. 'I just want to sleep. I'm just so tired of ... of ... of everything really. Everyone seems to know better than me what I should do, but, I don't know, don't want to hear them. Want some space. Want to ... I don't know what I do want anymore.' Dan sat looking at the floor. He looked heavy, weighed down. He was sniffing as if he had a cold, and looked a bit shaky.

'Sounds like you're in a bad way.'

Dan nodded and stared ahead of him. Jeannie watched him and waited. He had made the effort to be here, she thought, so that was a sign of something.

'I do stupid things. Fucking stupid.' He put his head in his hands, rubbed his face and yawned. As he lifted his hands up and away from his face he left his hair standing up at the front.

'Stupid things?' Jeannie sensed that Dan was moving towards telling her about what had happened. 'What do you mean?'

'Huh. Fucked up, didn't I? Thought it was a good idea at the time.' He shook his head.

'Mhmmm.' Jeannie waited.

'Tried to stop the meth.' He shook his head. 'I was so bloody determined. Just wanted to stop it ... but I couldn't, could I? Stupid thing to do.'

'Feels stupid now but at the time ... ?'

'At the time it felt right, I really wanted to do it, I really did. I've had enough of the drugs, I really have, I wanted to get clean, but I fucked up.'

'Yeah, I know how much you wanted to get clean, Dan, how you want to get off everything.'

Dan nodded. 'I tried, I really tried, I thought I could do it, thought I'd get through, thought I could stop. I don't know, I mean, I know you can't do that, deep down I know it, but that wasn't what was in my head on Friday.' He shook his head again; he was still looking at the floor. His hands were constantly moving, his fingers interlocking and then parting. He just looked so restless, so wound up by whatever had happened.

'Something else got into your head?'

Dan snorted. 'Something or someone: "the fucking addict". Bloody well took over again.'

'"The addict" made you stop?' Jeannie was curious as this seemed to be a bit of a contradiction at face value.

'Yeah, well, sort of, I don't know. Chaos in my head, that's what it was, chaos, but it seemed the right thing to do.' He looked up. 'I wanted to stop, you know that, and now it's all gone horribly wrong and I feel like fucking shit.'

'Yeah,' Jeannie paused, 'like fucking shit.'

> 'The addict' wanting him to stop is on the face of it strange, yet it is likely that this part would know he would not be able to stay off it and that it would generate chaos, which is part of the addict's raison d'être. It's like it used Dan's wish to be clean and the circumstance of the weekend to provoke an unrealistic attempt. For Dan, though, he was only able to engage with the idea that he was doing something reasonable and good, in memory of his brother. 'Parts' can be devious and manipulative, and this is a factor to consider, particularly parts that have developed out of drug use or are connected with it to some degree. The lengths people will go to for their next fix; the length 'parts' of ourselves will go to to gain satisfaction, in this case the satisfaction of re-establishing the prime identity of being a drug user – 'the addict' – and re-experiencing the introjected sense of chaos as normal and to be expected.

Dan sat with what he was feeling, which was a mixture of aches all over his body, a foggy head, and he just felt so heavy, so tired and worn out. He sat back in his chair and rocked his head back against the support, staring at the ceiling. He didn't speak for almost five minutes. Finally, he began to describe what had happened. 'I'd been thinking about Jake and, well, he died when he was nineteen and I'm twenty-nine and somehow I got to think it was the tenth anniversary of his death – on Sunday. I mean, I know now that it wasn't, that I just got my dates and everything all muddled up, but I thought it was the tenth anniversary of his death and it was when I was coming home Friday that I just knew I had to do something to kind of remember him by, wanted to make a statement of something. I don't know, but I got it into my head to stop the methadone. Didn't do anything then, but I was still thinking about it.'

'Mhmmm.' Jeannie did not want to interrupt the narrative.

'Went out to AA that evening. Just sat there. Wasn't really taking much in. Guess I was feeling kind of out of it, thinking about methadone and drugs and I guess I felt an outsider, you know, everyone talking about alcohol? I mean, you know I've drunk all my life until recently, and yeah, I've got a problem with it, which I thought I was dealing with, anyway, sat there and just felt so alone, so different. Just felt so bad. Usual stories, someone talked about being battered by his father and how he had drunk to forget how awful he felt and to get rid of the memories in his head. Said that it never had, he still had them but that he wasn't drinking any more. I remember thinking, yeah, that's me, and thinking about saying something but didn't want to admit to still using the meth. Just felt all wrong somehow. Just felt weird. Left straight after it finished.'

'Left feeling weird, yeah.'

'Yeah. Came straight home. Still thinking about Jake. Oh yeah, someone else had talked about his brother, how important he had been to him but how he had lost contact with him through drinking. Talked about how much he had loved him, and how much he missed him.' Dan snorted again and sighed. 'Did me the world of good, that did. So I left as soon as I could, came home, went upstairs, got the jar out of the bathroom cupboard and poured it down the sink. I remember thinking, here's to you Jake, no more of this fucking stuff, I'm gonna be clean for you on Sunday.'

'That's what you wanted, yeah, to be clean for Jake on his birthday.'

Jeannie gives a simple, direct empathic response to the focus that Dan has reached, allowing him to continue without disrupting his flow of thought and feeling.

'But I wasn't, well, not the meth. I was OK to begin with on Saturday, really thought I'd be OK. Went out with Gemma and her son, felt a bit edgy late morning, bit sweaty but thought it would pass. But I started to feel cramps by late afternoon, felt real bad. Told Gemma what I was doing. She was concerned but thought I knew what I was doing. So did I, but I knew I didn't. Set myself up. What was it I called that part of myself, oh yeah, "captain fucking chaos". Oh yeah, he came back on the scene with a vengeance that evening.'

'Chaos took over?'

Dan nodded. 'Gemma was concerned but I said I'd be OK. Said a few cans would settle me down for the night, I'd be OK then, just wanted to get through the night and then Sunday, just wanted to be clean for Jake, you know?' Dan shook his head. 'I loved that silly bastard, getting himself shot, or whatever happened.' Tears had welled up in his eyes and they were soon streaming down his face. 'Why did he have to fucking die, Jeannie, why? Some bastard shot him, I'm bloody sure of it, but we'll never know the truth now.'

Jeannie could feel the pain that was present in the room; she felt as if she could reach out and touch it. So much pain. Her lips tightened as she looked across at Dan, his head now back in his hands, his elbows on his knees.

'Why? It doesn't seem fair. Why? I tried to stay clean for him, Jeannie, I tried, I really tried. But I couldn't. I called a mate and he let me have some to get me through. I went and got some cans on the way home, strong lager and just went for it. Was I drunk. Shit. I was out of it, fucking rubber legs, could hardly stand, real mess. Don't remember much about getting home, but I did. Woke up on the settee, don't remember anything else. Gemma was furious. Said she had trusted me, that she couldn't anymore and that it wasn't going to happen again and if it did I was going to have to leave. Part of me wants to say, "fuck her then", but I know too that that isn't what I really want. She's been so good to me. I've got to get my head together, I really have.'

'Gemma's really important to you and part of you doesn't give a damn, yeah?'

Dan nodded, but said nothing. Yes, I know, I know, but it's down to me. I've got to get myself together, got to. He did not voice his thoughts.

Jeannie has responded to his mixed feelings towards Gemma, ignoring his recognition of his need to get his head together. He's only nodded rather than develop it further. It isn't what he wants to focus on, maybe too uncomfortable, maybe his sensed need to get his head together is far more present for him. Jeannie follows up by picking up on this.

'And you really want to get it together?'

Dan nodded again but looked so sad as he did so. He looked like that little boy again, so small and overwhelmed by it all. Somehow hearing Jeannie say what he was thinking and feeling was overwhelming. 'You suddenly look very small and so overwhelmed by what has happened.'

Dan took a deep breath. 'Yeah, but I can't stay like that. I've got to learn from this. Part of me feels, "what's the point?", but I know there is a point and I want to get back to earning Gemma's respect again. At least her son didn't see me; he had been dropped off at his grandmother's for the rest of the day and overnight. He doesn't need to see any of this.' He was shaking his head again. 'I have to try again. I've seen Marie. Spoke to her Monday. They've given me a script again and I'm under strict instructions not to do it again. They're right, of course. Said they thought I might need a slight increase but I said no, wanted to go back to 10 mls, but they have decided that I should be dispensed daily and that from now on any reduction is 1 ml at a time. But they want me to stabilise first, and they gave me a three-day supply of tranquillisers to help me make sure I stopped the alcohol. I appreciated that. I think otherwise I might have carried on, but I haven't. Last one of them tomorrow.'

'So, glad they gave you those, and you'll be back to just the 10 mls of methadone by Thursday?'

'Yeah. Hasn't been easy though, keep wanting to go to sleep. Am staying off sick till Thursday, that's my plan anyway. Just taking it slowly. Can't have too much time off; I don't like it but I need that job.'

Jeannie nodded. 'Yeah, the job's important however much it annoys you.'

'Very much. Just need to get stable again, you know?'

'Jeannie nodded. 'Yeah, be good to get stable again, get things on an even keel.'

Dan sat quietly for a moment. 'And I'm going to switch from AA to NA (Narcotics Anonymous). I think I needed AA initially, I think that was right, but I think I need to be with people who had similar drug experiences to me now. Not that I think I've sorted out the alcohol, but I think I need to get my priorities right. But I'll see how it goes. I haven't spoken to anyone yet, plan to do that tomorrow, phone around while I'm home and see what I can set up.'

'Seems timely, yeah, feeling you need that, I don't know, sort of commonality with other ex-drug users.'

'Yeah, but I'm not really an "ex" just yet, not while I'm still taking the meth. But I have to, and I've learned from last weekend. I won't do that again. And it wasn't the tenth anniversary of Jake dying anyway.' He shook his head. 'Crazy stuff. Really need to get myself together.'

This decision to switch to Narcotics Anonymous may be out of desperation. However, a profound shift may be occurring within his sense of self as he moves to perhaps accepting himself as a drug user and realising that he needs the company of other ex-users to help him move forward. His previously intense urge to be clean, to be free of the methadone might, in part, have also been connected to a sense of no longer wishing to own an identity of drug user as much as not wanting the chemicals in his body. However, it does not have to be *either* AA *or* NA; it can be both if that is what someone feels that they need.

Dan suddenly felt a coughing fit coming on; his throat had gone dry. He started coughing and couldn't seem to stop, making his eyes water. He couldn't clear his throat. Finally, after he had drunk a fair amount of water, it began to settle. 'Ohh.' He tried to clear his throat again; it still felt dry and tickly.

'Bit dehydrated?'

'Probably. Haven't drunk enough I guess. Nose has been running since Saturday. But I think it's easing now.'

The session continued with Dan talking about his feelings for Gemma, how good she was for him and how much he didn't want to mess that up as well. It was a sensitive topic and Jeannie felt deeply touched by how much feeling Dan was expressing for her, and she told him of this. This then affected him and left him being even more aware of his feelings for her. 'She kind of organises me. My mother never did, well, not like she does. But last weekend was out of control, out of her control and out of mine. Can't let it happen again.'

'You sound pretty clear about that.'

'Yeah. Can't quite understand what made me think I needed to be dry on Sunday for Jake, just got that into my head from somewhere. Already there before the meeting, got thinking that way at work, but don't know why.' Dan genuinely had no idea. Could have been any little thing.

'Something at work but you don't know why,' Jeannie replied, empathising with Dan's comment.

'Just a normal day. Spent a bit of time in the admin office, don't always do that, but I do from time to time. Something must have set me off. Didn't have those thoughts when I left home that morning.'

'Something after you left home?'

Dan thought. He wanted to know what it was. He really didn't want to be caught out again, but he remembered how they had identified 'the addict' and 'captain chaos' inside himself and he knew they were to blame, well, that meant he was to blame, of course.

'Jeannie, does it need a trigger, I mean, if there are parts of me that want to cause chaos and get me using, do they need a trigger? Or could they just kind of, I don't know, try to take over again?'

'Is that what you think might have happened?' Jeannie didn't answer his question as, to be quite honest, she didn't know the answer.

She had read about the idea of the self-concept fighting back (Mearns, 1992) and she knew that configurations could re-assert themselves, but did they need a trigger, or could Dan have just reached a point in himself where he had got bored with the normal life he was trying to create for himself? Somehow, that felt more realistic, but she wasn't at all sure. She knew how people who experienced a lot of disruption in early life could normalise it and find it very difficult to tolerate anything predictable, or devoid of risk, experiencing it as boring (Bryant-Jefferies, 2001).

'I don't know. I was kind of doing really well, I'd got into a new routine and getting to meetings and stuff, you know, it kind of felt good.'

'Mhmmm, felt good.'

'Yeah, it did. Felt like I was getting somewhere. Yeah . . .' Dan was remembering something and he went quiet as he thought about it. He had felt an urge to add something more, quite spontaneously as he had been speaking, but it had stopped him and left him thinking about it.

Jeannie did not know what Dan was thinking, but she did respond to what he had said, simply saying 'yeah?'in a slightly questioning manner, inviting Dan to share what he was thinking if he wanted to.

'Yeah, well, I was about to say, "like I wanted to celebrate".' He paused. 'Do you think that was what it was?'

'You wanting to celebrate?'

Yeah, well, sort of, but I could have celebrated, maybe that's not the right word, but somehow mark that thought of ten years since Jake's death, in some other way. Could have arranged to go out or something, didn't have to suddenly take it into my head to stop the meth and cause bloody cha-os.' Dan slowed down as he said the last work. 'Shit!' The word came out with some explosive force. 'Me wanting to celebrate got fucking hijacked.' He took a deep breath and blew it out.

'Maybe, hijacked by . . .?'

'"The addict" and "captain chaos". Yeah, oh yeah, that makes sense. Bastards. Yeah, they saw a fucking opportunity. Well, I'm getting wise to them and I'm not gonna fall for that one again.' He shook his head. 'Geez, I was pretty bloody devious in the past, you know, but those two.' He stopped again. 'But it's me, isn't it, I mean, it's me. It's my deviousness, they're just using it. Shit. I really have got to put the past behind me, haven't I?'

Jeannie nodded.

'OK, this is fucking war. That's what this is. War with me, with that fucking pair.' He blew out a breath. 'OK, well they had better make the most of my last few weeks of methadone 'cos they're gonna be without it soon.' Dan could feel more energy inside himself now, he could feel his motivation flowing back. 'Yeah, war, and they can threaten me with chemicals all they like, but I'm gonna fight back and create the life that I want. Yeah. What I want.'

Jeannie reflected her empathy for what Dan had concluded, using his own words so that he could hear them back. 'Fight back, create the life that I want.'

Dan was nodding.

Jeannie had noticed that time was nearly up. A thought was with her and she voiced it. 'We haven't much time now, but maybe that is something to really think about?'

'Yeah, I'll come back to that next week, Jeannie. I want to think about this, about what I do want. I kind of think I have more of a head full of what I don't want, but that's not enough. I want to have something positive to work towards. Yeah. I'm going to give this some thought and, yeah, maybe we can talk about that next week.'

'Sure.' They agreed the time and Dan left, feeling a lot more positive than when he had arrived. He was somewhat surprised how much he had changed. He seemed to have spent the whole lesson feeling bad about himself and then suddenly it all changed, and it seemed to have changed around him getting angry with 'the addict' and 'captain chaos'. Shit, he thought, am I mad? If I told people at work about these characters they'd lock me up! Maybe that's why I don't talk to them so much these days – the thought came at him like an instinctive reaction but it was a new insight for him. Yeah, he hadn't been saying too much recently. Maybe he didn't feel he had so much to say.

Jeannie was aware of feeling energised as well. Allowing Dan to stay with his feelings had somehow allowed him to make important recognitions for himself and to generate some strong feelings that he then seemed to be feeding off in a positive way. What a session. So much to talk about at her next supervision session later in the week, and then, well, see what Dan has in mind for his future life.

Points for discussion

- How do you see the role of anti-depressants and other mood-altering medication working in alliance with counselling? What problems might such medication pose to the therapeutic alliance?
- How do you react to a client spending so much time thieving to maintain a habit? How would being robbed or burgled yourself impact on your ability to work with such a client?
- Were you left after reading Session 18 with a sense that Dan was at some level preparing himself to just stop his methadone? What might you have said or done had you felt this?
- How were you left feeling or thinking after reading Session 19, and how did this contrast with your feelings and thoughts at the end of the previous session, or other sessions?
- Jeannie did not suggest that Dan could go to AA as well. What do you think was her theoretical rationale for this from a person-centred perspective?
- Dan has recognised that he is embarking on a chemical war inside his own body. It will have to be a war of attrition. Do you feel ready, willing and able to be a comrade with Dan in his personal war zone?

Summary

Dan talks of his lowering mood and discusses the possibility of anti-depressants. He becomes angry with himself that things are not changing enough for him; he wants to get off the methadone. Dan describes part of his past, the routine of stealing to get money for the gear, some of the incidents that occurred. He mentions that it would have been Jake's birthday next week. He talks more about his early drug use, his first use of tobacco and the feelings it gave him, the glue and the need for something stronger to get away from his memories of Billy and the crap at home. He reconnects with feelings of being tired of it all. Next session Dan describes how he stopped the methadone, poured it away, wanting to be clean in memory of Jake. He ends up drinking to try to stave off withdrawal and is given a short course of tranquillisers by Marie to get him off the alcohol. He is back on the methadone. Dan realises he has a chemical war on his hands – inside himself.

CHAPTER 12

Supervision 4

Jeannie had described to Max what had been happening since she had last seen him, and the struggle that Dan was having with himself, and with his current drug taking. How there had emerged within him a sense of not wanting to feel, that while he was motivated to change there seemed to be something working against it, and the wonder at the synchronicity of the flat battery, of wanting to get the methadone out of his system, get clean and sober and to move on to a new life.

'Mhmmm,' Max had listened with interest, 'so Dan is in quite a battle with himself?'

'At one point I'm sure he said something about it feeling like a war.'

'Mhmmm. And so he feels it's like a war; what about you?'

'What, how do I feel it is for him?'

'I was wondering more how it feels for you to be with him in the battle zone.'

Jeannie pondered for a moment, but in fact the answer had been a very swift, instinctive reaction. 'Shell-shocked.'

'Powerful experience, shell-shocked, can you describe it a little more?'

Jeannie stopped to think about it again. What did it feel like? She could try and be with as she felt now, but she knew that she wanted to connect with how it felt being with Dan, in the counselling room, in contact with him and his frame of reference. She thought back to recent sessions, but the last one stood out. The more she thought about it, the more she had a sense of just feeling overwhelmed by it all and a sense of being unsure where they were going. She recognised that in an intellectual sense she knew that theoretically it was a matter of offering the necessary and sufficient conditions and trusting the therapeutic process and the operation of the actualising tendency within Dan. She realised she had been thinking for a while and was aware of Max looking at her expectantly.

'Lost in thought. So many thoughts, Max. I mean, I know from a theoretical standpoint what I'm endeavouring to offer, and that gives me a frame of reference and kind of a sense of the whole process. And yet my actual experience of being with Dan is a sense of not really knowing what's going on around me, where I'm going, quite where I've been.' She stopped and a smile came across her face. 'Dazed and confused, wasn't that a song title?'

'I don't know, but it sounds like a good one. So that's how it leaves you feeling, dazed and confused.'

Jeannie nodded. 'I really don't know where we are going and I want to believe we are going somewhere, but I also know my job is to expect nothing and be Dan's companion in his inner world, but it isn't easy.'

'What isn't easy and how does it affect your offering the core conditions?'

'This sense of "anything can happen"; I mean, he has some pretty powerful configurations operating within him and there is a constant risk that he will lapse again.'

'And I'm interested in your use of language – that it is a risk. Maybe, though, he will need that experience still, that he isn't yet ready for sustainable change? Is it a risk when it is a need?'

'Meeting that need presents a risk to Dan, risk to his health, risk to his self-esteem which is already pretty low, risk to his relationship with Gemma, maybe his job. Yeah, he uses on top of his script now, or binges on alcohol into his "captain chaos" configuration, and anything can happen.'

'And that's really hard for you to be open to, the possibility of all of this.'

Jeannie realised that she wasn't accepting Dan as he was, that she was carrying hope for change, and strongly so. 'Maybe I'm not fully accepting of him, of the parts of him that could trigger some form of self-destruct.' She sat and reflected on this. 'I want him to come through all of this, Max.'

'I'm sure you do, and I'm sure parts of Dan do, but there are parts of him that are fearful of change, and which want to maintain the familiar, whatever the cost.'

Jeannie nodded. 'And maybe I'm not really hearing them or listening to them. They need to feel heard as well, don't they? They are as much part of Dan?'

Max nodded. 'This is the uniqueness of the person-centred approach, I think, that we offer unconditional acceptance to all aspects of our clients, not interfering, or trying not to, with our agenda and priority. That is the power of the approach?'

'I know, and I think I've lost sight of it. It's the drug-use culture. No, it's more the drug-service culture, you know? Harm reduction, harm minimisation. But some clients feel so bad about themselves that they want to harm themselves, or they know no different.'

The strategy of many drug services in the UK is primarily to reduce harm. This can take many forms and is not necessarily about stopping using. For instance, prescribing methadone as a substitute reduces harm; needle exchanges reduce harm; testing for infectious diseases and being vaccinated, for instance, against hepatitis B, can reduce harm; supporting people in changing risky patterns of use can reduce harm. Accepting that not everyone will want to stop using, but that their use can be changed such that the risk of harm is minimised, is an important attitude to inform service provision. Counselling can also be regarded as a harm-reduction strategy as it can offer the opportunity to resolve underlying difficulties that drive the drug use. The risk, however, is where difficult experiences, memories, come to the surface too quickly, leaving people at greater risk of lapsing back into their old patterns of use.

> The person-centred approach trusts that the person's own growth process will ensure that what is most pressing will come to the surface at a time when the person is ready to deal with it. However, reduced drug use can affect this, causing memories to emerge quite forcefully from behind the chemical barrier. Hence the need at times for other medication to be used to help people through this difficult transition, while at the same time the client is being offered the opportunity to experience the healing potency of the therapeutic relationship based on person-centred principles and values.

'And how does that part get heard, the part that wants to do harm?'

'Well, often it doesn't, or it only does when the person does harm to themselves.' Jeannie hadn't actually thought that through but as she heard herself say the words she was shocked, and yet felt that there was a truth in them. 'That's quite shocking, isn't it?'

'You feel shocked?'

'Yeah, I mean, I wonder how often the person is really allowed to reveal that side of themselves, I mean really talk about it? Drug workers are so sensitive to risk and harm minimisation that perhaps they don't allow that part to be heard; they seek to problem solve or emphasise the positive to motivate them not to do harm, but that could be a collusion, couldn't it?'

'Collusion?'

'Colluding to keep the part that wants to do harm silent, but it won't stay silent, will it? It'll find a way of emerging and often to devastating and destructive effect.'

'OK, so where does this lead you to insofar as your relationship with Dan?'

Jeannie paused. 'I think I am listening to the part of him that wants to cause chaos.' She stopped again. 'But then, in fact the part of him that seems more present is what he calls "the addict". I don't know that "captain chaos" has ever really made any kind of directly verbal expression to me. He stays silent and yet he drives it all. He's not speaking, is he? He's not getting heard. Am I stopping him from being heard? Am I refusing to listen, to really listen to and to hear that part of him?' Jeannie was aware that this line of thought had really taken her aback. She wasn't sure. 'I'm not sure, Max, but I think I need to be more sensitive to it somehow, listen for it communicating in some way.'

'So, this rather shadowy part of himself doesn't openly communicate, but it does seem to trigger off certain behaviours that can be destructive?'

'Yes, but I've always assumed to simply produce the experience of chaos for Dan, what he's kind of "normalised". Don't think I like that word, I mean, it sounds judgemental and I don't want to be that way, but it is what has been introjected – an "I am chaotic" introject which he has to live up to.'

Max nodded. 'So where does this leave you?'

'I'm not sure how much I am open to hearing this.' Jeannie was aware that her heart felt as if it was racing a little. Anxiety, she thought, so something is going on for me here. 'My heart's racing. There is something anxiety making here for me.'

> Here again is evidenced the value of supervision and the importance of the supervisee allowing their experiencing to be open and transparent within the supervisory relationship.

' "I am chaotic" causing anxiety?' Max realised as he said it that it was him putting two and two together. 'That may just be me putting two and two together, and may not be as it is.'

Jeannie could feel the anxiety spreading. 'I need to stay with this. I'm getting a stronger reaction here.' She could feel her arms getting sort of heavy but 'nervy' feeling, like a subtle tickle in her muscles. She closed her eyes and tried to relax her way into her physiological experience. Nothing, but her heart was pounding. She continued to stay with it. She knew that there was something and it needed to surface. It was blocking her and she needed to clear it if she was to be able to genuinely hear that part of Dan that was not only chaotic but potentially self-destructive.

Max waited, allowing Jeannie the space to be in her own process. He had felt his own senses sharpen and knew that he needed to be focused and sensitive to whatever emerged for Jeannie, and be open to the possibility that it might not emerge at this time.

Chaos. Self-destruct. Jeannie held these words in her mind while seeking to be open to all that was present for her. She suddenly felt very weak as feelings rapidly emerged, overwhelming feelings that took her back to her brother's death and the chaos at home. And she remembered that one afternoon, a wet Sunday it was, she was on her own and didn't know what to do. She felt so lost without him, and no one seemed to be coping well. She suddenly recalled, as vivid as if it was happening, how she had sat there looking out of the window for some time thinking that perhaps she would be better off dead as well. She had talked about it before in therapy and she thought she had dealt with it, but it was now very present for her.

'It's me, fear of my own self-destruction. Something I thought I had dealt with in therapy but it's still there and Dan has brought it to the surface.' She explained her thoughts and feelings to Max, who nodded and affirmed that he had heard her, and that he wondered what she felt she needed to do.

Jeannie felt it needed to go back to therapy; she needed to raise it and work with it once more. 'Do these experiences ever go away, or do they emerge when we work with certain people and we then need to re-engage with that aspect of ourselves elsewhere to help us keep ourselves clear?'

'I don't think things are always once-and-for-all dealt with. I think we hope to know ourselves well enough to know when we are reacting from within ourselves in such a way that we may be compromising our offering of empathy, unconditional positive regard, congruence and a sense of contact with the client. And we have supervision so that hopefully it gets recognised and can be addressed because these are the kinds of internal reactions that we can miss, that in effect part of us wants to miss to preserve our own sense of ease or well-being.'

'They make us uncomfortable and we don't like to be uncomfortable, but as therapists we have to override that and be prepared to sit in the discomfort zone in ourselves to be with our clients.'

Max nodded. 'If we cannot sit with our own discomfort we won't be much good sitting with our client's.'

'It's a therapy issue, not a supervision issue. If I try and deal with it here I think it will take up too much time. But I do want to keep it on the agenda here to check out its impact on my work. It would be really helpful if you could keep this in the back of your mind.' Jeannie paused. 'Stupid request.'

'Yeah, it'll be in the forefront, has to be, first duty is to ensure the client is safe. We are talking about part of Dan that is self-destructive. It needs to be heard. You need to be able to hear it.'

'And if I can't, well, I need to be open with him about it.'

'It may come to that. For now it needs monitoring.'

Jeannie nodded. 'OK. Thank goodness I have you to talk to. So many other professions just don't have this space for processing personal reactions to clients and yet they offer some kind of listening skills to clients. Many even call it counselling. It's scary, particularly working with this client group where their whole way of life can sometimes be built around a self-destructive tendency.'

'It is scary. I don't feel at ease with it. I think the risk is that some people with self-destructive tendencies can feel unheard; the part of them that doesn't want to harm themselves is heard, and is engaged with through risk assessments and harm reduction strategies, but who listens to the part that embodies the urge to self-destruct? Yes, it is uncomfortable to listen to and, in an increasingly legislative climate, professionals can get very anxious.'

'And the self-destructive part that has developed perhaps from some traumatic episode or reinforcement over a number of years remains without a voice and an opportunity to be understood.'

'No different to any other part of ourselves, just needs to be heard and in that process of being heard, feeling accepted and understood, it can begin to become more integrated within the person and less differentiated, less intense and therefore less likely to trigger behaviour.' Max paused. 'OK, we've got away from the specifics of yourself and Dan. I think it is important that this has arisen and, yes, it does need addressing in therapy as you have recognised and I will be mindful of it in our work. And no doubt you will be more aware of it too with Dan?'

Jeannie nodded. 'At times it feels like a constant process for the counsellor as much as for the client, and of course it is!'

'I often think of an image that I think Rogers used somewhere, the notion of seeing himself as being a bit like a mirror for the client to see themselves in, and that his job was to keep the mirror clean so the image of themselves that the client sees is not obscured by misty or murky bits of the therapist!'

'I need to clean my mirror. Maybe that's how it is. We clean off the smudges, but it isn't a once-and-for-all clean. Like any mirror, we have to keep it clean. It can get smudged again, in the same place or in other places. Yes, I like that idea. I've got a smudge on chaos and self-destruct in my mirror. It needs a therapeutic clean.'

CHAPTER 13

Dan reflects on his goals for the future

Session 20

Jeannie was very aware of the discussion in her last supervision session and had had a therapy session since then and begun to address the chaos and self-destruct issues in her self. It had been very helpful. Yes, it did feel as though her mirror had got smudged again. The sense she was left with was that it's as though that bit of the glass gets damaged and somehow, as a result, smudges tend to stick and build up quicker than elsewhere. It probably wasn't just working with Dan that had exacerbated the smudge; it may already have been building up without her realising it. Anyway, she was addressing it now and she had an image that she would certainly carry with her. She was aware of smiling to herself. Such a simple image, and yet so much meaning and value to it.

She walked into the waiting room, still pursuing her train of thought.

'Hi, Jeannie.' Dan stood up in the waiting room as Jeannie entered. He had noticed the smile on her face. He was glad she looked pleased to see him, particularly after the last session and what had preceded it.

'Hi, Dan. Come on through.' Jeannie turned and walked back to the counselling room, Dan following her. They sat down.

'So, how do you want to use our time today, Dan? I know we discussed a possible focus at the end of the last session, but there may be something more pressing for you.'

'Yeah. I've been giving it a lot of thought, and I do want to think about the future, and how I get there. I have stabilised again. Bit rocky last week, but things have settled. I'm having another week on the 10 mls and then reducing 1 ml per week, and I am going to be getting it in the appropriate doses per day, so that will help. So it means that in about ten weeks' time, all being well, I'll be clear of it. At least that's what I want to work towards. I know there are a lot of assumptions in this, but that's my goal as far as that is concerned.'

Jeannie nodded. 'And you feel good about this planned reduction?'

'Yeah, I do. It feels controlled somehow, but I have to watch that I don't get some daft idea in my head again. But, well, I hope that won't happen.'

> This gradual process will probably involve Dan developing a configurational part within his Self that allows him to experience this as being satisfying. In a real sense, the actual adaptation he must make within himself to sustain this is itself a therapeutic spin-off.

'Yeah, I hope so too.' Jeannie felt she wanted to convey her own feelings to Dan, but she added as well, 'But if a problem arises we'll explore it and hopefully learn from it.'

'It's good to feel that if I do slip up again that at least I can come and explore it. Marie feels the same way. I don't get a sense that I'll somehow be judged, although I know I'll judge myself.'

'Judge yourself?'

'I can be really critical of myself when I don't do what I plan to do. I mean, it's like if no one else condemns me then I step in and condemn myself.'

'So a part of you really condemns you for not doing what you plan to do.'

Dan nodded. 'Like there's a kind of critical bit of me, little voice somewhere telling me that there I go again, not got it right, or not reached your goal. It always has a certain tone to it and reminds me of my father who was always critical of me, telling me I was good for nothing. Part of me wants to prove him wrong.'

'Mhmmm, part of you wants to prove that your father was wrong.'

'Yeah.' But as Dan replied he knew there was another part of him that believed what his father had told him so many times. 'But there's this critical part of me that tells me I'm useless, good for nothing and won't achieve anything. That part depresses me at times.'

'Depressed at the thought of being good for nothing . . .'

'Pisses me off, and yet it's so familiar too, like I've carried this around with me for so long.'

> Sounds like another configuration, Jeannie thought, but said nothing, knowing that she needed to maintain her empathy with Dan and not drift into her own speculations and theorising. She was also aware that this critical part constrasted with the more 'what the hell' attitude that had been explored in an earlier session.

'So you've carried this critical part of you around for a long time, and it pisses you off.'

Dan nodded.

'Really pisses you off.'

'Yeah, fucking does. And yet what have I achieved? Years of drugs, no real career prospects, chaos in my head, all my friends are drug users and my main social life seems to be centred around going to meetings.'

Jeannie nodded. 'Doesn't feel like you have achieved much.'

'No, well I haven't, have I?'

'That's the way it is for you, and it gets to you.' Jeannie added the last bit, observing Dan's tightening jaw.

'Fucking does. I know I've got a chance of something new with Gemma, and I really want that to work out, but what have I done with my life up till now? Fuck all.'

'Mhmmm, fuck all.'

Jeannie stays with Dan, not trying to rescue him from his negative view of himself and his life, but consistently letting him know that she is hearing what he is saying. She does not offer him an alternative view; her role as a person-centred counsellor is to stay within his frame of reference, trusting that his own process will take him to where he needs to be and that this will have a constructive effect.

Dan heard Jeannie respond and he thought, yeah, fuck all. Hearing it just sums it all up. And he knew he wanted to change but he just didn't know how or what to do. He wanted things to change quicker than they seemed to be, and he also knew that that wasn't the answer either. The thoughts spun around in his head leaving him not knowing what to say or think.

Jeannie stayed with the silence. Dan looked as if he was thinking or feeling about what he had just been talking about. She trusted that whatever was happening within Dan would prove helpful and so she sought to maintain her focus and an attitude of warm acceptance, and waited for him to speak.

'I feel so stuck sometimes. I want to change, I want things to be different, and yet it's so hard and I can't always really get a sense of what I want. I mean, I know I want things to be different, but, I mean, I'm not sure exactly what I do want.'

'Like you know what you don't want but not what you do want?' As soon as she said it Jeannie realised that she had introduced an idea of her own, and yet the sentence had just flowed from her so easily and instinctively that she also felt that maybe she needed to trust this.

Sometimes responses are made without a sense of whether they are appropriate. Jeannie and Dan are on their twentieth session, the relationship will have developed and it is likely therefore that Jeannie will be much more tuned in to Dan. This can have the effect of the counsellor responding empathically to the client in ways that are reflective of what is present for the client even though the client may not have communicated it. Nevertheless, there will also be occasions when the counsellor says something instinctively and it is not related to the client; it is not something emerging out of their increased sensitivity towards the client's way of being, but will simply be a reflection of something present within the counsellor relating back to their own experiences. Even when this is the case, though, it can end up being helpful as the client may choose to reject what the counsellor has said, which helps them clarify what they really do mean.

'I'm not sure I know anything. I just want to be, to feel, well, different, feel I'm . . . yeah, feel I'm going somewhere. Not just taking it one day at a time, but feel I want a goal, something to aim for, something to work towards.'
'A goal to work towards, yeah, something longer-term?'
'Yeah.' Dan paused, aware of a fear inside himself. 'I don't want the chaos.'
Jeannie felt herself react and was aware of heightening her concentration. 'That sounds affirming – you don't want chaos.'
'No. And I know I don't want the drugs. But it's hard to say what I do want. I mean, chaos, drugs, been part of my life for so long. I want to be different, really different, but I don't know what. I see people, married, mortgages, kids, good jobs, yeah, and I want to be like that, at least I think I do, but that also feels like a huge jump, I mean a really huge jump. It's like, yeah, nice idea, but I can't see it happening to me. It's like I can't really see beyond how I've been and I guess,' Dan sighed, 'I guess the truth is that even if I did have these things I'd be shit-scared of losing them, of messing up, and I'd feel a hundred times worse than I do now.'
'That's one hell of a scary thought: get what you want but mess up and lose it and feel much worse than you do now.'
'It would be so easy, I feel really vulnerable to everything going pear-shaped.'
'Yeah, it sounds hugely vulnerable.'
Dan went quiet. Yeah, he did feel vulnerable, and he knew that other part of him seemed to feel invincible so long as everything was in chaos. He knew that it was the chaotic part of himself that put him at risk of doing himself damage, and yet he knew he survived in chaos. 'But the chaotic me feels invincible.'
Jeannie noted that the chaotic side was being described and she was ready to hear it. 'Yeah, you feel invincible in the chaos.'

Prior to the last supervision session, Jeannie could have found herself offering Dan the choice of exploring either the vulnerable or the chaotic, invincible part. And this could even have been done in a way that would subtly direct Dan back to the vulnerable part and lose the opportunity of engaging with the dangerous, chaotic bit. A response of 'so part of you feels invincible, but another really vulnerable' would have left the emphasis on the vulnerability, would have been directive and would most likely have emerged from Jeannie's own incongruence. Now, however, she is able to respond directly to what Dan has said, and maintain focus in his current frame of reference.

'Yeah, I do. I can cope with chaos, I always have, I thrive on it, feel good in it, it's me, what I do best. What the hell, live for the day, get your buzz, fuck everyone else, yeah.'

'Sounds really alive, full of thrills and excitement.' Jeannie was aware that she was trying to engage now specifically with this part of Dan that thrived on chaos. She really wanted it to feel heard. She was also aware of how fast Dan had switched into this part of himself. She guessed that this configuration was very much self-contained and perhaps this aspect of it had been encouraged by the chemical impact of the drug use that was associated with it.

'Yeah, and I have survived. Lot of people around me haven't, but I have. Yeah, I take risks, but that's part of it. Makes me feel good.'

'I can hear that. Risks feel really, really good.'

'Yeah. Yeah, they do.'

'So, you plan to keep on taking risks, yeah, maintain the buzz, live the chaos?'

'Yeah, I do.' Dan paused and frowned. 'What am I saying here? No. I can't go on like this, it'll kill me, or mess me up for good.'

'Mhmmm, that's part of the risk.'

'Yeah, part of the risk, and I can feel part of me wants to say, "great, risks", but I don't want to say that.'

'You don't want to say that, but part of you does.'

'Yeah, me that takes risks with myself, causes chaos. It's a powerful part of me but I need to replace it with something else. I need to grow into an alternative to it.'

'So an alternative, what, something really different?'

Dan thought about it and somehow, while that seemed reasonable, he wasn't sure. 'Seems like I need to take risks but make it safer somehow.'

'You mean take safer risks?'

Take safer risks. That was an interesting thought. Was that what he was saying? Yes, it was, the more he thought about it, yes, that was what he needed. But what would it mean? 'Yeah, I mean, maybe I could keep this risky chaotic me but seek something different for it to focus on?'

'You mean something dangerous but somehow with some kind of built-in safety?'

'Yeah, like, I don't know, something like parachuting or white-water rafting or something. Or maybe it doesn't have to be extreme, but something with a thrill, an edge to it. That might be enough. I mean, I don't know, but something rather than just try and get rid of it altogether.'

'Mhmmm, so do something that has a safe risk to it, a thrill, an edge so that you can allow that part of your nature to live out but without it being too dangerous, too chaotic?'

'Something like that. I think it's something to go and think about.' Dan paused. 'But I think I want to be off the meth first.'

'OK, but it is something to work towards.'

'Yeah. Yeah, I really need to think about this. I need something to get into, you know, something different but with some excitement.' As he sat and thought he realised that there was something else he needed to do as well. 'I also need to get fit. I mean, I know what I do at work is quite manual, but maybe I need to do some fitness stuff. That could be quite a buzz. Maybe we could all do that,

Gemma as well. Get her mother to look after her son one evening a week or something. Yeah, I'll suggest that.'

'Sounds like you are having some ideas now as to what you do want in your life.'

'I need something that isn't bland. That's where I think I've gone wrong. Doing stuff around the house is OK, and so is going to meetings, but I want to work towards more than that, or at least alternatives. But I've got to get off the meth as well. Though maybe I could still start at the gym. There's one in the local leisure centre I think. Maybe Gemma could take her son as well, we could all do things.'

'Sounds really positive, something you can encourage each other with.'

'But I have to make it happen, don't I? Down to me.' Dan stopped and reflected. 'There is a way out of all of this, isn't there, but it isn't going to be easy. I'm going to have to make fresh choices and find ways to satisfy the parts of myself that previously got what they needed out of the drugs and the lifestyle I developed around using.'

'Yes, fresh choices to satisfy those parts of you.'

'And I am aware that I'm still going to feel kind of uncertain for a while I guess, uncertain whether I can hold it together. But I won't know unless I try.'

'Yes, that uncertainty will be around, but, yes, unless you try . . .'

Dan tightened his lips and nodded. 'Yeah, OK, there is some stuff to work for here. I'm going to give it a go.'

'Mhmmm, sounds strong and affirming. You're going to give it a go.'

Dan realised he felt stronger than that. 'No, it's going to happen. I need a fresh start. I'm not going to change overnight. I have to learn to be me but in a way that puts me and the people and things that are important to me at less risk. I'm clear on that.'

'Mhmmm, learn to be a you that does not put people and things that are important to you at risk.'

'I need to find that "me", become that "me".' Dan looked at Jeannie. 'I guess I've started. I guess that's what all this is about. And I guess I have a long way to go. So many years of . . . of . . . crazy years. Some good, but most of it not, not really, although at the time, well, different story. But I can't keep dwelling on it. It happened. I am where I am today and must accept it but also try to change it as well.'

'Yeah, accept it and change it, become that "me" that you seek to be.' Jeannie tried to reflect something of the gist of what Dan had said but avoid repeating it all back to him.

'Yeah, the drug use, the chaos, the stuff from my past, yeah, it happened, it all happened, but that was then and I've got to let it go, find new ways to be me, and that's like scary.'

'Scary stuff.'

'Yeah, but exciting too. Yeah, maybe that sense of excitement is important as well. I think I've been only considering sort of routine, mundane things to do, and that hasn't worked and I don't think it will work.'

Jeannie agreed and voiced her agreement. She knew, as well, that people changed and that maybe in time Dan would find himself more able to tolerate the routine stuff of life.

Dan continued. 'It's about me, isn't it? It's about me making choices, fresh choices, choices not driven by my past, by being messed up as a child and with the drugs and stuff, but choices driven by me as an adult taking responsibility for my life.'

Funnily, he looked as if he had grown a little in the chair as he had been speaking. She shared this. Maybe it was some weird indication that, yes, he was growing up.

The session drew to a close. Jeannie was left feeling positive for Dan and pleased with the way she felt she had handled the sessions and particularly in hearing the part of Dan that thrived on chaos and risk to himself. But she also knew there was a long way to go and that ahead of him there could, and probably would, be pitfalls. She knew that resolving not just drug use but also the underlying issues and behaviours associated with it would take time. But she had plenty of that. Counselling was open-ended.

She didn't feel so dazed and confused as she had last week. Something had shifted inside her. She wasn't sure what, but clearly beginning to address her own sensitivity to chaos and self-destruction was timely. She knew she would need to keep working on herself, that was part of being a person-centred counsellor. Yes, she hoped Dan would be able to create a lifestyle that was fulfilling and satisfying to himself and that he would not need the recourse to drugs in the future. She felt she had developed a good working relationship with him and that he trusted her. The next ten weeks would be critical as he slowly reduced the methadone. It was a long time but she hoped that he would redirect his frustration into other activities during that time. She was pleased he had switched to NA. She knew he would get support and encouragement and would feel perhaps more free to talk about his drug use.

Jeannie hoped Dan would keep off the alcohol, at least for some while. He might decide to try for controlled drinking later, but that wasn't something they had discussed and it could wait until such time as Dan might be thinking about it. Some people who used alcohol problematically had to remain abstinent, but there were others who, on resolving underlying issues, and for whom the heavy drinking had not been over a prolonged and substantial period of their life, could sustain control. Anyway, that was the future. For now, Dan had to get through his methadone reduction and begin to build a new life for himself. She felt good to be part of his process.

Yes, being a counsellor could take you through every possible feeling under the sun, expose you to insights and experiences that pushed your warm acceptance of the client to the limit and leave you feeling as if your emotions had been spun in a washing machine. But she still came back for more, knowing that the sense of having helped someone through recovery made it all worthwhile.

And Dan? He left the session more determined than ever to make changes and prepare himself for a new life. He felt he was getting to know himself better. Yes, that lapse the previous week had been stupid and he needed to watch for crazy ideas in his head. He knew he couldn't be complacent. He had described it as war and it was war, a chemical war, a biological war, call it what you will, but it was a war with himself. Yes, he was determined. He didn't know what lay ahead but he knew he had started a journey into a future that, while the actual content was uncertain, he was determined to ensure was not like his past. Drugs? He'd survived them, just. Many hadn't and don't. He was lucky. Yeah, maybe I am lucky, he thought as he sat in the car on the way home. Maybe there is hope for me. He glanced across at Gemma. He felt lucky. He felt a warm glow in his heart and a lump came to his throat. Yeah, he thought, I've got some good things to live for. He felt himself smile, and his eyes had watered. 'I love you, Gemma, you're good for me, and it's time I started being good for you.' He turned the radio on. It was a report on the news. There was some guy talking at some peace rally in London. 'Keep hope alive. Keep hope alive,' he was calling to the crowd. 'I need some of that,' Dan said out loud. Yeah, there's hope, Dan thought, and I'm gonna keep it alive in me.

Points for discussion

- How are you left feeling after reading this counselling session?
- Do you feel optimistic or pessimistic about Dan's future, and why?
- What were the key moments within the counselling process for Dan?
- What aspects of your own nature might make it difficult for you to work with Dan?
- Do you feel that Jeannie consistently applied a person-centred approach to counselling?
- How significant a part did supervision play in the therapeutic process?
- Contrast your attitude towards drug users and working with drug users at the start of reading this book with that which you are now experiencing.

Summary

Dan talks of his methadone-reduction plan and his acceptance of this. He describes feeling how little he has achieved in his life and how critical he can be of himself, which he sees linked back to his father's attitude towards him. He describes his feelings of being stuck, but also of his need for a goal, a direction. He realises how scary and risky change is, and how much change there has to be both in himself and in his lifestyle. He realises he has choices.

Author's comments

In writing this book I have become aware of an addictive aspect to myself. I noticed how it left me becoming so focused on the writing that other aspects of life were becoming ignored and not dealt with. I had so tuned into 'the addict' in myself, perhaps we all have one to a greater or lesser extent, that I was spending every free moment, and some that should not have been free, adding more dialogue. It became virtually the centre of my life for a few weeks.

In a sense, this was extremely helpful. It certainly offered me insights about myself. But it also showed me how easy it is to become absorbed in something, particularly a something that has an addictive element or interest within it. So, I too entered into a form of parallel process, discovering that Dan's configurations were affecting my own life. It has helped me appreciate how, when we work with our clients in a genuinely deeply therapeutic way, we are going to be profoundly affected and we need supervision to unravel ourselves from the relationship we have formed.

Of course, not all counselling goes to this depth. Yet it does not always require depth for a profound effect to be made upon the therapist. So the importance of regular supervision that embraces both personal and professional support, growth and development are vital components in effective counselling.

This book has not been able to cover every issue that Dan may have. His experiences in prison have not been dealt with, not to any great extent, and it may be that he has no issues with it, or it may arise later in the counselling process. Clients can take time to disclose certain experiences, sometimes years. His use of cocaine has not been a major feature of the therapeutic counselling here described. His relationships with his family remain sketchy: mother, his living brother and his father who no longer drinks.

I hope that this book has offered insight into this area of work. Not all recovering drug users will be like Dan; everyone is unique, everyone has their own problems and everyone will work at their own pace. Dan entered counselling at a time when his drug use was being brought under control. Yes, he had lapses, but that is part of the process of change (Bryant-Jefferies, 2001). Other drug-using clients will be more chaotic from the start, or more ambivalent about the whole process, being more devoted to maintaining their drug use, just wanting the problems to go away without the pain and effort of change.

In our society, drug users are often presented as social problems, inadequates, criminals and no-hopers. Well, I don't believe that this is a helpful perspective.

Drug users are first and foremost people, like the rest of us, living with the consequences of life experiences and the choices that they have made. Like most of us, change is often difficult to contemplate, made harder where an addictive substance is involved. But people can and do grow out of drug use, or make changes to their use such that they can achieve stability and avoid harm to themselves, or others.

It is my hope that in writing this book I will have helped you to help those who, for whatever reason, have got caught up in problematic drug use and wish to do something about it.

References

Advisory Council on the Misuse of Drugs (1998) *Drug Misuse and the Environment*. Home Office, HMSO, London.

Bailey AA (1974) *The Consciousness of the Atom* (2e). Lucis Press Ltd, London. Originally published in 1922.

Bedor C (2002) Counselling people recovering from drug addiction. In: K Etherington (ed.) *Rehabilitation Counselling in Physical and Mental Health*. Jessica Kingsley Publishers, London.

Bozarth J (1998) *Person-Centred Therapy: a revolutionary paradigm*. PCCS Books, Ross-on-Wye.

Bozarth JD and Wilkins P (eds) (2001) *Rogers' Therapeutic Conditions: evolution, theory and practice. Volume 1: Unconditional Positive Regard*. PCCS Books, Ross-on-Wye.

Bryant-Jefferies R (2001) *Counselling the Person Beyond the Alcohol Problem*. Jessica Kingsley Publishers, London.

Bryant-Jefferies R (2002) Rehabilitating the problem drinker in the community. In: K Etherington (ed.) *Rehabilitation Counselling in Physical and Mental Health*. Jessica Kingsley Publishers, London.

Carr A (2002) *A Handbook of Child and Adolescent Clinical Psychology*. Brunner-Routledge, Hove. Originally printed in 1999 by Routledge, London.

Gaylin N (2001) *Family, Self and Psychotherapy: a person-centred perspective*. PCCS Books, Ross-on-Wye.

Haugh S and Merry T (eds) (2001) *Rogers' Therapeutic Conditions: evolution, theory and practice. Volume 2: Empathy*. PCCS Books, Ross-on-Wye.

Mearns D (1992) On the self-concept fighting back. In: W Dryden (ed.) *Hard Earned Lessons from Counselling in Action*. Sage, London.

Mearns D (2000) The nature of 'configurations' within self. In: D Mearns and B Thorne (eds) *Person-Centred Therapy Today*. Sage Publications, London.

Mearns D and Thorne B (1988) *Person-Centred Counselling in Action*. Sage, London.

Mearns D and Thorne B (1999) *Person-Centred Counselling in Action* (2e). Sage, London.

Mearns D and Thorne B (2000) *Person-Centred Therapy Today*. Sage Publications, London.

Merry T (2002) *Learning and Being in Person-Centred Counselling* (2e). PCCS Books, Ross-on-Wye.

Rogers CR (1957) The necessary and sufficient conditions of therapeutic personality change. *Journal of Consulting Psychology*. 21: 95–103.

Rogers CR (1959) A theory of therapy, personality and interpersonal relationships as developed in the client-centred framework. In: S Koch (ed.) *Psychology: a study of a science. Volume 3: Formulations of the Person and the Social Context.* McGraw-Hill, New York, pp. 219–35.

Rogers CR (1961) *On Becoming a Person.* Constable, London.

Rogers CR (1980) *A Way of Being.* Houghton-Mifflin Company, Boston, MA.

Rogers CR (1986) A client-centered/person-centered approach to therapy. In: I Kutash and A Wolfe (eds) *Psychotherapists' Casebook.* Jossey Bass, San Francisco, CA.

Ross CA (1999) Subpersonalities and multiple personalities: a dissociative continuum. In: J Rowan and M Cooper (eds) *The Plural Self.* Sage, London, pp. 183–97.

Society for the Study of Addiction (1999) *Tackling Alcohol Together: a pre-publication summary.* Free Association Press, London.

Tyler A (1995) *Street Drugs: the facts explained, the myths exploded* (3e). Hodder and Stoughton, London. First edition published in 1986.

Warner M (2000) Person-centred therapy at the difficult edge: a developmentally based model of fragile and dissociated process. In: D Mearns and B Thorne (eds) *Person-Centred Therapy Today.* Sage Publications, London.

Warner M (2002) Psychological contact, meaningful process and human nature. In: G Wyatt and V Sanders (eds) *Rogers' Therapeutic Conditions: evolution, theory and practice. Volume 4: Contact and Perception.* PCCS Books, Ross-on-Wye.

Wyatt G (ed.) (2001) *Rogers' Therapeutic Conditions: evolution, theory and practice. Volume 1: Congruence.* PCCS Books, Ross-on-Wye.

Wyatt G and Sanders P (eds) (2002) *Rogers' Therapeutic Conditions: evolution, theory and practice. Volume 4: Contact and Perception.* PCCS Books, Ross-on-Wye.

Further reading

Bryant-Jefferies R (2003) *Problem Drinking: a person-centred dialogue*. Radcliffe Medical Press, Oxford.

Lockley P (1995) *Counselling Heroin and Other Drug Users*. Free Association Books Ltd, London.

Lowinson JH, Ruiz P, Millman RB and Langrod JG (eds) (1997) *Substance Abuse: a comprehensive textbook* (3e). Williams and Wilkins, Baltimore.

Owen L (1991) *What's Wrong With Me: breaking the chain of adolescent co-dependency*. Deaconess, London.

Pagliaro A and Pagliaro L (1996) *Substance Use Among Children and Adolescents*. Wiley, New York.

Plant M and Plant M (1992) *Risk-Takers: alcohol, drugs, sex and youth*. Routledge, London.

Stanton M and Todd T (1982) *The Family Therapy of Drug Abuse and Addiction*. Guildford Press, New York.

Szapocznik J and Kurtines W (1989) *Breakthroughs in Family Therapy with Drug Abusing Youth*. Springer, New York.

Useful contacts

Drugs

Adfam
Support to families and friends of drug users
Tel: 020 7928 8898
Website: www.adfam.org.uk

Drugscope
Membership organisation serving professionals in the field
Tel: 08707 743 682
Email: info@drugscope.org.uk
Website: www.drugscope.org.uk

Narcotics Anonymous (NA)
Tel: 020 7730 0009

National Drugs Helpline
Tel: 0800 776600
Website: www.ndh.org.uk

National Treatment Agency for Substance Misuse (NHS)
Tel: 020 7972 2214
Email: nta.enquiries@nta.gsi.gov.uk
Website: www.nta.nhs.uk

Re-Solv
The Society for the Prevention of Solvent and Volatile Substance Abuse
Email: information@re-solv.org
Website: www.re-solv.org

Release
Legal advice for drug users
Tel: 020 7729 5255
Email: info@release.org.uk
Website: www.release.org.uk

Person-centred

Association for the Development of the Person-Centered Approach (ADPCA)
Email: adpca-web@signs.portents.com
Website: www.adpca.org

An international association, with members in 27 countries, for those interested in the development of client-centred therapy and the person-centred approach.

British Association for the Person-Centred Approach (BAPCA)
Bm-BAPCA
London WC1N 3XX

Tel: 01989 770948
Email: info@bapca.org.uk
Website: www.bapca.org.uk

National association promoting the person-centred approach. Publishes the journal *Person-Centred Practice* and a regular newsletter *Person-to-Person*.

Person Centred Therapy Scotland
Tel: 0870 7650871
Email: info@pctscotland.co.uk
Website: www.pctscotland.co.uk

An association of person-centred therapists in Scotland which offers training and networking opportunities to members, with the aim of fostering high standards of professional practice.

World Association for Person-Centered and Experiential Psychotherapy and Counselling
Email: secretariat@pce-world.org
Website: www.pce-world.org

Index